COLORADO CAMPGROUND LOCATOR MAP

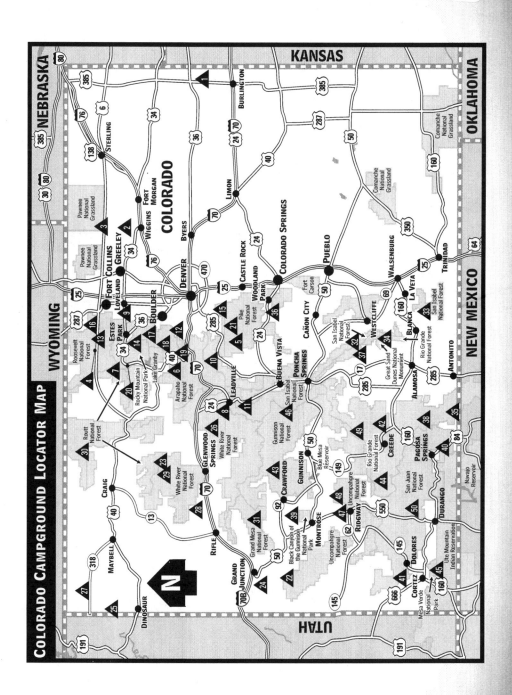

MAP LEGEND

WHITE WOLF
Campground name
and location

Individual tent and RV
campsites within
campground area

TABLE ROCK
Group campsites
or other nearby
campgrounds

NATIONAL FOREST **STATE PARK**
Public lands

⟨**64**⟩ Interstate highways

⟨**19**⟩⟨**219**⟩ US highways

⟨**325**⟩⟨**219**⟩⟨**SR-219**⟩
State County Service
roads roads   roads

MAIN ST.
Other roads

Unpaved or
gravel roads

Boardwalk

Political
boundary

+++++++
Railroads

– – – – –
Hiking, biking,
or horse trail

SWIFT CREEK
River or stream

ASHEVILLE
◉
City
or town

N
Indicates North

WARD LAKE
Ocean, lake,
or bay

Bridge or tunnel	Playground	Picnic area
Amphitheater	Parking	Sheltered picnic area
Falls or rapids	Marina or boat ramp	Spring/well
Food	Fire ring	Dishwater disposal
Restroom	Telephone	Summit or lookout
Water access	Laundry	Bathhouse
Gate	Cemetery	Dump station
Trash	Swimming	No swimming
Wheelchair accessible	Horse trail	Stables
Hospital/medical care	Postal dropoff	Ranger office

OVERVIEW
MAP KEY

EASTERN COLORADO

1 BONNY LAKE STATE PARK CAMPGROUND
2 JACKSON LAKE STATE PARK
   CAMPGROUND
3 PAWNEE NATIONAL GRASSLAND
   CAMPGROUND

NORTH CENTRAL COLORADO

4 BROWNS PARK CAMPGROUND
5 BUFFALO CAMPGROUND
6 BYERS CREEK CAMPGROUND
7 THE CRAGS CAMPGROUND
8 ELBERT CREEK CAMPGROUND
9 FLATIRON RESERVOIR CAMPGROUND
10 GENEVA PARK CAMPGROUND
11 GOLD PARK CAMPGROUND
12 GOLDEN GATE CANYON STATE PARK
   CAMPGROUND
13 JACKS GULCH CAMPGROUND
14 LONGS PEAK CAMPGROUND
15 LOST PARK CAMPGROUND
16 LOWER NARROWS CAMPGROUND
17 PEACEFUL VALLEY AND CAMP DICK
   CAMPGROUNDS
18 RAINBOW LAKES CAMPGROUND
19 ROBBERS ROOST CAMPGROUND
20 TIMBER CREEK CAMPGROUND
21 WESTON PASS CAMPGROUND

NORTHWEST COLORADO

22 BIG DOMINGUEZ CAMPGROUND
23 COLD SPRINGS CAMPGROUND
24 COLORADO NATIONAL MONUMENT:
   SADDLEHORN CAMPGROUND
25 DINOSAUR NATIONAL MONUMENT:
   ECHO PARK CAMPGROUND

26 FULFORD CAVE CAMPGROUND
27 IRISH CANYON CAMPGROUND
28 RIFLE FALLS STATE PARK CAMPGROUND
29 SHEPHERDS RIM CAMPGROUND
30 STEAMBOAT LAKE STATE PARK
   CAMPGROUND
31 WEIR AND JOHNSON CAMPGROUND

SOUTH CENTRAL COLORADO

32 ALVARADO CAMPGROUND
33 BEAR LAKE CAMPGROUND
34 GREAT SAND DUNES NATIONAL
   PARK AND PRESERVE: PINYON FLATS
   CAMPGROUND
35 MIX LAKE CAMPGROUND
36 MUELLER STATE PARK CAMPGROUND
37 NORTH CRESTONE CREEK CAMPGROUND
38 TRUJILLO MEADOWS CAMPGROUND

SOUTHWEST COLORADO

39 BLACK CANYON OF THE GUNNISON
   NATIONAL PARK: NORTH RIM
   CAMPGROUND
40 BLANCO RIVER CAMPGROUND
41 BURRO BRIDGE CAMPGROUND
42 CATHEDRAL CAMPGROUND
43 LOST LAKE CAMPGROUND
44 LOST TRAIL CAMPGROUND
45 MESA VERDE NATIONAL PARK:
   MOREFIELD CAMPGROUND
46 MIRROR LAKE CAMPGROUND
47 RIDGWAY STATE PARK
   CAMPGROUND
48 SILVER JACK CAMPGROUND
49 STONE CELLAR CAMPGROUND
50 TRANSFER PARK CAMPGROUND

Other Books by Kim Lipker

60 Hikes within 60 Miles: Denver and Boulder
The Unofficial Guide to Bed and Breakfasts and Country Inns in the Rockies
Day & Overnight Hikes: Rocky Mountains National Park (2008)

Other Books by Johnny Molloy

Backcountry Fishing: A Guide for Hikers, Paddlers, and Backpackpackers
Beach and Coastal Camping in Florida
Beach and Coastal Camping in the Southeast
The Best in Tent Camping: The Carolinas
The Best in Tent Camping: Florida
The Best in Tent Camping: Georgia
The Best in Tent Camping: Kentucky
The Best in Tent Camping: The Southern Appalachian and Smoky Mountains
The Best in Tent Camping: Tennessee
The Best in Tent Camping: West Virginia
The Best in Tent Camping: Wisconsin (with Kevin Revolinski)
Canoeing & Kayaking Florida (with Liz Carter)
Canoeing & Kayaking Guide to Kentucky (with Bob Sehlinger)
Day & Overnight Hikes: Great Smoky Mountains National Park
Day & Overnight Hikes: Kentucky's Sheltowee Trace
Day & Overnight Hikes: Shenandoah National Park
Day & Overnight Hikes: West Virginia's Monongahela National Forest
Exploring Mammoth Cave National Park
50 Hikes in the North Georgia Mountains
50 Hikes in the Ozarks
50 Hikes in South Carolina
From the Swamp to the Keys: A Paddle through Florida History
Hiking the Florida Trail: 1,100 Miles, 78 Days, and Two Pairs of Boots
The Hiking Trails of Florida's National Forests, Parks, and Preserves (with Sandra Friend)
Land Between the Lakes Outdoor Recreation Handbook
Long Trails of the Southeast
Mount Rogers Outdoor Recreation Handbook
A Paddler's Guide to Everglades National Park
60 Hikes within 60 Miles: Austin and San Antonio (with Tom Taylor)
60 Hikes within 60 Miles: Nashville
Trial by Trail: Backpacking in the Smoky Mountains

Visit Johnny Molloy's Web site:
www.johnnymolloy.com

THE BEST IN TENT CAMPING

A GUIDE FOR CAR CAMPERS WHO HATE RVs, CONCRETE SLABS, AND LOUD PORTABLE STEREOS

COLORADO

FOURTH EDITION

Kim Lipker and Johnny Molloy

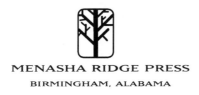

MENASHA RIDGE PRESS

BIRMINGHAM, ALABAMA

For John Bland, who got it all started. —JM

Copyright © 2007 by Johnny Molloy

All rights reserved

Printed in the United States of America

Published by Menasha Ridge Press

Distributed by the Publishers Group West

Fourth edition, second printing 2010

Library of Congress Cataloging-in-Publication Data

The best in tent camping, Colorado : a guide for car campers who hate RVs, concrete slabs, and loud portable stereos. -- 4th ed. / Kim Lipker and Johnny Molloy.

p. cm.

Rev. ed. of: Best in tent camping, Colorado / Johnny Molloy. 3rd ed. 2004.

Includes bibliographical references and index.

ISBN-13: 978-0-89732-645-2 (alk. paper)

ISBN-10: 0-89732-645-8 (alk. paper)

1. Camping—Colorado—Guidebooks. 2. Camp sites, facilities, etc.—Colorado—Guidebooks. 3. Colorado—Guidebooks. I. Lipker, Kim, 1969– II. Molloy, Johnny, 1961– III. Molloy, Johnny, 1961– Best in tent camping, Colorado.

GV191.42.C6M65 2007

917.88'068--dc22

2007017800

Cover and text design by Ian Szymkowiak, Palace Press International, Inc.

Cover photo by J. C. Leacock/Alamy

Cartography by Steve Jones and Johnny Molloy

Indexing by Galen Schroeder

Menasha Ridge Press

P.O. Box 43673

Birmingham, Alabama 35243

www.menasharidge.com

TABLE OF CONTENTS

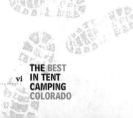

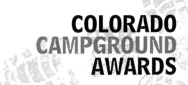

COLORADO CAMPGROUND AWARDS

ACKNOWLEDGMENTS

I WOULD LIKE TO THANK THE FOLLOWING PEOPLE who helped with the fourth-edition update: Johnny Molloy, Bruce Becker, Russell Helms, Molly Merkle, Karen Lipker, Abby Balfany, Jen Janssen, Darcy Blaisdell, Alex, Anna, and Emma Lipker; Ruth and Roger Lipker; Diane Stanko and Marty Martinez; and finally, the helpful folks at the National Park Service, the USDA Forest Service, and the Colorado State Parks.

—Kim Lipker

THANKS TO THE FOLLOWING FOR their help with the original editions of the guide: Joe Mayer, Sam Berry, Becky Anderson, Kate Brannan, Paul Welschinger, Susan Webster, Margaret Albrecht, Bryan Delay, James Herbaugh, Pat Molloy, Bill Armstrong, Keith Stinnett, Bryan Hatfield, Michael and Nan Wolfenbarger, Nelle Molloy, Larry of Castle Rock; Beverly, Wilbert, and Craig Spieker of Castle Rock, who made me feel at home; Regi Roberts, John Cox, and David Zaczyk, master of the semicolon.

—Johnny Molloy

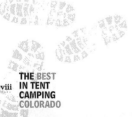

PREFACE

OH, WHAT A JOY IT WAS TO RESEARCH THIS BOOK! In the beginning, the task of finding the 50 best campgrounds in Colorado seemed daunting, for there are hundreds of campgrounds located among the millions of acres of national- and state-forest land, national parks and monuments, and other public lands. But the months of exploring Colorado's varied landscape turned into a journey through a scenic wonderland. The Rockies come to mind first, where craggy, snow-covered mountains tower over verdant meadows, cool alpine lakes reflect deep forests and cobalt skies, and snow-fed mountain streams crash down narrow valleys. But there are other sides of Colorado: the amazing cliff dwellings of Mesa Verde, the chasm of the Black Canyon of the Gunnison, the alluring reservoirs of the plains, the immense Great Sand Dunes backed against the Sangre de Cristo Range, the white water of the Arkansas River, the red-rock country of the Uncompahgre Plateau, and more.

After seeing this tremendous variation, I wanted the reader to be able to combine enjoying these sights and with having a quality camping experience at a good campground. I toured the state's natural and historic features by day, then typed up on-site reports from the nearby camps where I stayed, using a computer powered by my car battery.

Each day's experience left me looking forward to the next day, to see if I could find campgrounds to match the beauty of the landscape. Spells of cold and rain and wrong turns and long drives to campgrounds that failed to make the book could not overwhelm the sense of awe I felt while surveying the real Colorado. The subject material overwhelmed the actual physical process of finding the best campgrounds. In other words, researching Colorado was a blast!

And it can be for you, too, pitching your tent at 3,500 feet in the plains or 12,000 feet in the mountains, and just about every elevation and situation in between. Here, you can relax in attractive settings. Beyond the campgrounds you can hike canyons, climb "fourteeners," raft wild rivers, fish remote trout streams, mountain bike tabletop mesas, boat reservoirs, go caving, and recall Colorado's history. Combine this book and a slice of your precious time, then do a little exploring of your own.

—Johnny Molloy

A NOTE ABOUT THE FOURTH EDITION

Revising something that is otherwise perfect is both an honor and a daunting task. I was approached as a Rocky Mountain expert to update existing profiles, delete old campgrounds, and add new ones. We also reorganized the book according to more commonly known regions (around these parts, at least), refined the maps, and wrote a more thorough introduction to tent camping—all while keeping the same friendly tone and accuracy for which Johnny Molloy is known. We hope you'll like the changes, and we encourage you to get out and find your favorite "room with a view" in Colorado.

—Kim Lipker

ABOUT THE AUTHORS

JOHNNY MOLLOY IS AN OUTDOOR WRITER based in Johnson City, Tennessee. Born in Memphis, he moved to Knoxville in 1980 to attend the University of Tennessee. During his college years, he developed a love of the natural world that has since become the primary focus of his life.

It all started on a backpacking foray into the Great Smoky Mountains National Park. That first trip was a disaster; nevertheless, Johnny discovered an affinity for the outdoors that would lead him to backpack and canoe-camp throughout the United States over the next 25 years. Today, he averages 150 nights out per year.

After graduating from UT with a degree in Economics, Johnny spent an ever-increasing amount of time in the wild, becoming more skilled in a variety of environments. Friends enjoyed his adventure stories; one even suggested that he write a book. He pursued that idea and soon parlayed his love of the outdoors into an occupation.

The results of his efforts are more than 40 books. These include hiking, camping, paddling, and other comprehensive guidebooks, as well as books on true outdoor adventures. Johnny has also written for numerous publications and Web sites. He continues to write and travel extensively to all four corners of the United States, exploring a variety of outdoor activities. For the latest on Johnny, please visit **www.johnnymalloy.com.**

KIM LIPKER GREW UP IN COLORADO loving the outdoors from an early age. She is the author of two other guidebooks for Menasha Ridge Press, *Day & Overnight Hikes in Rocky Mountain National Park* and *60 Hikes within 60 Miles: Denver and Boulder.* She also wrote *The Unofficial Guide to Bed & Breakfasts and Country Inns in the Rockies* (Hungry Minds). In addition to writing books, Kim writes a regular parenting column and other features for *Rocky Mountain Parent Magazine;* for the Web site Away.com, she contributes features, ratings, and reviews covering parks, active sports, and outdoor adventures in the Rocky Mountains and Hawaii.

Considered an expert on the Rocky Mountains by her guidebook peers, Kim has been at the writing thing for a while, having had her first news article published at age 12 and later earning a journalism degree from the University of Missouri–Columbia.

Kim lives in Fort Collins, Colorado, with her three children, Anna, Alex, and Emma. For more information on her upcoming projects, visit her blog at **trekalong.com/lipker.**

THE BEST IN TENT CAMPING

A GUIDE FOR CAR CAMPERS WHO HATE RVs,
CONCRETE SLABS, AND LOUD PORTABLE STEREOS

COLORADO

FOURTH EDITION

INTRODUCTION

WELCOME TO THE FOURTH EDITION of *The Best in Tent Camping Colorado.* If you're new to tent camping or even if you're a seasoned camper, take a few minutes to read the following introduction. We explain how this book is organized and how to use it.

THE OVERVIEW MAP AND OVERVIEW–MAP KEY

Use the overview map on the inside front cover to assess the exact location of each campground. The campground's number appears not only on the overview map but also on the map key facing the overview map, in the table of contents, and on the profile's first page.

The book is organized by region as indicated in the table of contents. A map legend that details the symbols found on the campground layout maps appears on the inside back cover.

CAMPGROUND–LAYOUT MAPS

Each profile contains a detailed campground layout map that provides an overhead look at campground sites, internal roads, facilities, and other key items. Each campground entrance's GPS coordinates are included with each profile.

GPS CAMPGROUND–ENTRANCE COORDINATES

This book includes the GPS coordinates for each campground entrance in two formats: latitude–longitude and UTM. Latitude–longitude coordinates tell you where you are by locating a point west (latitude) of the 0° meridian line that passes through Greenwich, England, and north or south of the 0° (longitude) line that belts the Earth, aka the Equator.

Topographic maps show latitude–longitude as well as UTM grid lines. Known as UTM coordinates, the numbers index a specific point using a grid method. The survey datum used to arrive at the coordinates in this book is WGS84 (versus NAD27 or WGS83). For readers who own a GPS unit, whether handheld or onboard a vehicle, the latitude–longitude or UTM coordinates provided on the first page of each profile may be entered into the GPS unit. Just make sure your GPS unit is set to navigate using WGS84 datum. Now you can navigate directly to the campground.

However, readers can easily find all campgrounds in this book by using the directions given and the campground layout map, which shows at least one major road leading into the area. But for those who enjoy using the latest GPS technology to navigate, the necessary data has been provided. A brief explanation of the UTM coordinates from Flatiron Reservoir Campground (page 39) follows on the next page.

```
UTM Zone (WGS84)    13T
Easting   0480500
Northing  4468900
Latitude   N 39° 55' 10"
Longitude  W 105° 40' 40"
```

The UTM zone number 13 refers to one of the 60 vertical zones of the Universal Transverse Mercator (UTM) projection. Each zone is 6 degrees wide. The UTM zone letter T refers to one of the 20 horizontal zones that span from 80 degrees South to 84 degrees North. The easting number 0480500 indicates in meters how far east or west a point is from the central meridian of the zone. Increasing easting coordinates on a topo map or on your GPS screen indicate that you are moving east; decreasing easting coordinates indicate you are moving west. The northing number 4468900 references in meters how far you are from the equator. Above and below the equator, increasing northing coordinates indicate you are traveling north; decreasing northing coordinates indicate you are traveling south. To learn more about how to enhance your outdoor experiences with GPS technology, refer to *GPS Outdoors: A Practical Guide for Outdoor Enthusiasts* (Menasha Ridge Press).

THE CAMPGROUND PROFILE

In addition to maps each profile contains a concise but informative narrative of the campground, as well as individual sites. This descriptive text is enhanced with at-a-glance ratings and information, GPS-based trailhead coordinates, and accurate driving directions that lead you from a major road to the parking area most convenient to the trailhead. On the first page of each profile is a ratings box.

THE RATING SYSTEM

This book includes a rating system for Colorado's 50 best tent campgrounds. Six campground attributes—beauty, privacy, spaciousness, quiet, security, and cleanliness—are ranked using a five-star system. A low rating in one or two areas, especially privacy and spaciousness, was not necessarily grounds for exclusion from this book. In some cases, the nature of the terrain just doesn't allow for big, private sites, yet the campground still may be well worth a visit. This system should help you find what you are looking for.

BEAUTY In judging beauty, we took into account both what the general area has to offer as well as the campground. The most beautiful campgrounds have sites that you just don't want to leave and locations with easy access to breathtaking scenery.

PRIVACY Privacy is determined by how much your neighbors can pay attention to what you are doing and you to what they are doing. The best campgrounds have plenty of green space (shrubs and trees) between adjoining sites, as well as staggered sites (that is, the entrance to the site across the road is not directly opposite yours).

SPACIOUSNESS While this category contributes to the amount of privacy you have, it refers mostly to how much space you have to move around in. The sites at some campgrounds are surprisingly large—to the point of overkill; others are incredibly small.

QUIET Our evaluations were influenced to a great extent by the presence of RVs and the kinds of visitors a park tends to get (campgrounds near urban areas, for example, usually are a bit noisy, as are those that cater to families with children). We also considered the extent to which you could get away from the fray at a particular campground. You can expect some variation within my ratings based on whether you visit a campground during the week or on a weekend; on holiday weekends, all bets are off.

SECURITY With few exceptions, we've found Colorado campgrounds to be very safe and secure, due largely to the presence of campground hosts and park rangers making the rounds. The only places at which we felt security might be compromised were those remote campgrounds that saw few visitors and had no host or ranger on duty.

CLEANLINESS Our judgments were based on the presence and remnants of past campers around the campsite (trash, tent stakes, burned logs, etc.) and on the restroom facilities. We did take into account that primitive toilets tend to be a little less tidy than modern facilities, although there seemed to us to be little reason for either to be a mess.

WEATHER

We must stress that the weather in Colorado can change every ten minutes. Be prepared for anything: sun, snow, flash flood, lightning, and hail. Start by knowing the weather forecast and the road conditions; then pack smart. It can be a lovely day in Denver, but a campground may be inaccessible due to blizzard conditions. You must be prepared, and you should consider carrying a hiking card (CORSAR, discussed on the next page). If you need to be rescued, these cards can save your life and your pocketbook.

ROAD CONDITIONS
Colorado Traffic Management Center
of CDOT
www.cotrip.org
(877) 315-7623

AVALANCHE WARNINGS
Colorado Avalanche Information Center
www.geosurvey.state.co.us/avalanche
(303) 499-9650

CLIMATE OVERVIEW
Semiarid
Dry summers
Short springs
Mild winters except in the mountains

MEAN TEMPERATURE BY MONTH: DENVER AREA

	JAN	FEB	MAR	APR	MAY	JUN
HIGH	43	47	52	62	71	81
LOW	16	20	26	35	44	52

	JUL	AUG	SEP	OCT	NOV	DEC
HIGH	88	86	77	66	53	45
LOW	59	57	48	36	25	17

It is hard to generalize the climate and the altitude throughout Colorado but we can tell you that what you pack and how you deal with the altitude can make or break a camping trip.

The Rockies' rugged and varied geography creates a number of weather zones. Whatever the region, whatever the season, be sure to dress in layers. In the summer, expect warm days and cool evenings. Bring shorts, hiking boots, a sweater, and a weatherproof jacket. In the winter, bring snow gear for the mountains and warm outerwear for elsewhere.

ALTITUDE SICKNESS Nothing ruins an outing more often than the body's resistance to altitude adjustment. The illness is usually characterized by vomiting, loss of breath, extreme headache, lightheadedness, sleeplessness, and an overall sick feeling. Our advice: take it easy. When traveling to a higher altitude, give your body a day or two to adjust to where there is less oxygen, hotter sun, and less air pressure. Drink plenty of water, and lay off the alcohol and cigarettes. Wear sunglasses and sunscreen. It's that easy. (As always, if serious symptoms persist, locate the nearest emergency room or call 911.)

LIGHTNING AND TORNADOES Violent storms are common in June, July, and August. If you are caught in a lightning storm above treeline, stay off ridgetops, spread out if you are in a group and squat or sit on a foam pad with your feet together. Keep away from rock outcroppings and isolated trees. If someone has been struck, be prepared to use CPR to help restore breathing and heartbeat.

In the event of a tornado (they are extremely common in the eastern portion of Colorado) immediately seek shelter. If you are in an open field, lie down in the nearest ditch.

CORSAR

The Colorado Outdoor Recreation Search and Rescue Card (CORSAR) may be purchased at most outdoor shops, such as REI. You can buy a one-year card for $3 or spend $12 and buy a five-year card. CORSAR is not insurance—it does not pay for medical transportation, which may include helicopter flights or ground ambulance. The card does allow reimbursement to county sheriffs for costs included on a mission. These expenses can include mileage, meals, equipment, gasoline, and rental fees (horses, ATVs, aircraft) for vehicles used in the search. It says right on the CORSAR information that "you have helped ensure that trained and well-equipped search and rescue teams will respond should you become lost or in need of rescue and they will not have to incur undue expense due to your emergency."

FIRST-AID KIT

A typical first-aid kit may contain more items than you might think necessary. These are just the basics. Prepackaged kits in waterproof bags are available (Atwater Carey and Adventure Medical make a variety of such kits). As a preventive measure, take along sunscreen and insect repellent. Even though there are quite a few items in the following list, they do pack down into a small space:

Ace bandages or Spenco joint wraps

Antibiotic ointment (Neosporin or the generic equivalent)

Aspirin or acetaminophen

Band-Aids

Benadryl or the generic equivalent, diphenhydramine (in case of allergic reactions)

Butterfly-closure bandages

Epinephrine in a prefilled syringe (for people known to have severe allergic reactions to such things as bee stings)

Gauze (one roll)

Gauze-compress pads (a half-dozen 4- x 4-inch pads)

Hydrogen peroxide or iodine

Matches or pocket lighter

Moleskin/Spenco "Second Skin"

Whistle (it's more effective in signaling rescuers than your voice)

ANIMAL AND PLANT HAZARDS

BLACK BEARS There are no definite rules about what to do if you meet a bear. In most cases the bear will detect you first and leave. If you do encounter a bear, here are some suggestions from the National Park Service:

- Stay calm.
- Move away, talking loudly to let the bear discover your presence.
- Back away while facing the bear.
- Avoid eye contact.
- Give the bear plenty of room to escape; bears will rarely attack unless they are threatened or provoked.
- Don't run or make sudden movements; running will provoke the bear and you can not outrun a bear.
- Do not attempt to climb trees to escape bears, especially a black bear. The bear will pull you down by the foot.
- Fight back if you are attacked. Black bears have been driven away when people have fought back with rocks, sticks, binoculars, and even their bare hands.
- Be grateful that it's not a grizzly bear.

MOUNTAIN LIONS Lion attacks on people are rare, with fewer than 12 fatalities in 100 years. Based on observations by people who have come in contact with mountain lions, some patterns are beginning to emerge. Here are more suggestions from the National Park Service:

- Stay calm.
- Talk firmly to the lion.
- Move slowly.

- Back up or stop; never run because lions will chase and attack.
- Raise your arms. If you are wearing a sweater or coat; open it and hold it wide.
- Pick up children and make them appear larger.
- If the lion becomes aggressive, throw rocks and large objects at it. This is the time to convince the lion that you are not prey and that you are a danger to them.
- Never crouch down, or turn your back to retrieve said items.
- Fight back and try to remain standing if you are attacked.

TICKS Ticks like to hang out in the brush that grows around campsites and along trails. Their numbers seem to explode in the hot summer months, but you should be tick-aware during all months of the year. Ticks, which are arthropods and not insects, need a host to feast on in order to reproduce. The ticks that light onto you will be very small, sometimes so tiny that you won't be able to spot them. Primarily of two varieties, deer ticks and dog ticks, both need a few hours of actual attachment before they can transmit any disease they may harbor. Ticks may settle in shoes, socks, hats, and may take several hours to actually latch on. The best strategy is to visually check yourself a couple of times a day, especially if you've gone out for a walk in the woods. Ticks that haven't attached are easily removed, but not easily killed. If you pick off a tick in the woods, just toss it aside. If you find one on your body at camp, you may want to dispatch it (other-wise, it may find you again). For ticks that are embedded, removal with tweezers is best.

RATTLESNAKE

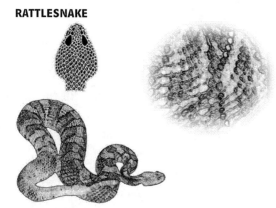

SNAKES Spend some time in Colorado and you may be surprised by the variety of snakes in the area. Most snake encounters will be with garter snakes, water snakes, and bull snakes (while not venomous, they are rather large and scary look-ing). The only venomous snake in the region is the rattlesnake. Rattler sightings are very common. A good rule of thumb is to give rattlers a wide berth and leave them alone. In the chance that you are bitten by a rattlesnake stay calm and get help immediately.

POISON IVY Recognizing poison ivy and avoiding contact with it is the most effective way to prevent the painful, itchy rashes associated with these plants. In the West, poison ivy is found as a small plant with three leaflets to a leaf. Remember "leaves of three, let them be." Urushiol, the oil in the sap of these plants, is responsible for the rash. Usu-ally within 12 to 14 hours of exposure (but sometimes much later), raised lines and/or blisters will appear, accompanied by a terrible itch. Refrain from scratching because bacteria under fingernails can cause infection and you will spread the rash to other parts of your body. Wash and dry the rash thoroughly, applying calamine lotion or another product to help dry the rash. If itching or blistering is severe, seek medical attention. Remember that oil-contaminated clothes, pets, or hiking gear can easily cause an irritating rash on you or someone else, so wash not only any exposed parts of your body but also clothes, gear, and pets.

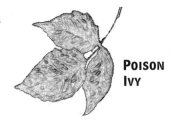

POISON IVY

MOSQUITOES Although it's not a common occurrence, individuals can become infected with the West Nile virus by being bitten by an infected mosquito. Culex mosquitoes, the primary variety that can transmit West Nile virus to humans, thrive in urban rather than natural areas. They lay their eggs in stagnant water and can breed in any standing water that remains for more than five days.

Most people infected with West Nile virus have no symptoms of illness, but some may become ill, usually 3 to 15 days after being bitten. In Colorado, August and September are the high-risk periods for West Nile virus. At this time of year—and anytime you expect mosquitoes to be buzzing around—you may want to wear protective clothing such as long sleeves, long pants, and socks. Loose-fitting, light-colored clothing is best. Spray clothing with insect repellent. Remember to follow the instructions on the repellent carefully, and take extra care with children.

TIPS FOR A HAPPY CAMPING TRIP

There is nothing worse than a bad camping trip, especially since it is so easy to have a great time. To assist with making your outing a happy one, here are some pointers:

- **RESERVE YOUR SITE AHEAD OF TIME,** especially if it's a weekend, a holiday, or if the campground is wildly popular. Many prime campgrounds require at least a six-month lead time on reservations. Check before you go.

- **PICK YOUR CAMPING BUDDIES WISELY.** A family trip is pretty straightforward, but you may want to consider including grumpy Uncle Fred who does not like bugs, sunshine, or marshmallows. After you know who is going, make sure that everyone is on the same page regarding expectations of difficulty, sleeping arrangements, and food requirements.

- **DON'T DUPLICATE EQUIPMENT** such as cooking pots and lanterns among campers in your party. Carry what you need to have a good time, but don't turn the trip into a major moving experience.

- **DRESS APPROPRIATELY FOR THE SEASON.** Educate yourself on the highs and lows of the specific area you plan to visit. It may be warm at night in the summer in your backyard, but up in the mountains it will be quite chilly.

- **PITCH YOUR TENT ON A LEVEL SURFACE** preferably one that is covered with leaves, pine straw, or grass. Pitch your tent on a tarp or specially designed footprint to thwart ground moisture and to protect the tent floor. Do a little site maintenance such as picking up small rocks and sticks that can damage your tent floor and make sleep uncomfortable. If you have a separate tent rain fly but don't need it, keep it rolled up at the base of the tent in case it starts raining at midnight.

- **IF YOU ARE NOT USED TO SLEEPING ON THE GROUND,** take a sleeping pad with you. Take one that is full-length and thicker than you think you might need. This will not only keep your hips from aching on hard ground, but will also help keep you warm.

- **IF YOU ARE NOT HIKING INTO A PRIMITIVE CAMPSITE,** there is no real need to skimp on food due to weight. Plan tasty meals and bring everything you will need to prepare, cook, eat, and clean up the mess.

- **IF YOU'RE PRONE TO USING THE BATHROOM MULTIPLE TIMES AT NIGHT,** you should plan ahead. Leaving a warm sleeping bag and stumbling around in the dark to find the rest room, whether it be an outhouse, a fully plumbed facility, or just the woods, is second best. Keep a flashlight and any other accoutrements you may need by the tent door and know exactly where to head in the dark.

- **STANDING DEAD TREES AND STORM-DAMAGED LIVING TREES** can pose a real hazard to tent campers. These trees may have loose or broken limbs that could fall at any time. When choosing a spot to rest or a backcountry campsite, look up.

CAMPING ETIQUETTE

Camping experiences can vary wildly depending on a variety of factors such as weather, preparedness, fellow campers, and time of year. Here are a few tips on how to create good vibes with fellow campers and wildlife you encounter.

- **OBTAIN ALL PERMITS AND AUTHORIZATION AS REQUIRED.** Make sure you check in, pay your fee, and mark your site as directed. Don't make the mistake of grabbing a seemingly empty site that looks more appealing than your site. It could be reserved. If you are unhappy with the site you've selected, check with the campground host for other options.

- **LEAVE ONLY FOOTPRINTS.** Be sensitive to the ground beneath you. Be sure to place all garbage in designated receptacles or pack it out if none is available. No one likes to see the trash someone else has left behind.

- **NEVER SPOOK ANIMALS.** It's common for animals to wander through campsites, where they may be accustomed to the presence of humans (and our food). An unannounced approach, a sudden movement, or a loud noise startles most animals. A surprised animal can be dangerous to you, to others, and to themselves. Give them plenty of space.

- **PLAN AHEAD.** Know your equipment, your ability, and the area in which you are camping—and prepare accordingly. Be self-sufficient at all times; carry necessary supplies for changes in weather or other conditions. A well-executed trip is a satisfaction to you and to others.

- **BE COURTEOUS TO OTHER CAMPERS,** hikers, bikers, and others you encounter. If you run into the owner of a large RV, don't panic. Just wave, feign eye contact, and then walk away slowly.

- **STRICTLY FOLLOW THE CAMPGROUND'S RULES** regarding the building of fires. Never burn trash. Trash smoke smells horrible and trash debris in a fire pit or grill is unsightly.

BACKCOUNTRY-CAMPING ADVICE

Be sure to check if a permit is required before entering the backcountry to camp and always strive to practice low-impact camping. Adhere to the adages "Pack it in, pack it out," and "Take only pictures, leave only footprints." Practice "leave no trace" camping ethics while in the backcountry.

Open fires are permitted except during dry times when the Forest Service may issue a fire ban. Backpacking stoves are strongly encouraged. You are required to hang your food from bears and other animals in order to minimize human impact on wildlife, avoid their introduction to and dependence on human food. Wildlife learns to associate backpacks and backpackers with easy food sources, thereby influencing its behavior. Make sure you have about 40 feet of thin but sturdy rope to properly secure your food. Ideally, you should throw your rope over a stout limb that extends ten or more feet above ground. Make sure the rope hangs at least five feet away from the tree trunk.

Solid human waste must be buried in a hole at least three inches deep and at least 200 feet away from trails and water sources; a trowel is basic backpacking equipment.

Following the above guidelines will increase your chances for a pleasant, safe, and low-impact interaction with nature.

VENTURING AWAY FROM THE CAMPGROUND

If you go for a hike, bike, or other excursion into the boondocks, here are some tips:

- **ALWAYS CARRY FOOD AND WATER** whether you are planning to go overnight or not. Food will give you energy, help keep you warm, and sustain you in an emergency situation until help arrives. You never know if you will have a stream nearby when you become thirsty. Bring potable water or treat water before drinking it from a stream. Boil or filter all found water before drinking it.

- **STAY ON DESIGNATED TRAILS.** Most hikers get lost when they leave the path. Even on the most clearly marked trails, there is usually a point where you have to stop and consider which direction to head. If you become disoriented, don't panic. As soon as you think you may be off-track, stop, assess your current direction, and then retrace your steps back to the point where you went awry. If you become absolutely unsure of how to continue, return to your vehicle the way you came in. Should you become completely lost and have no idea of how to return to the trailhead, remaining in place along the trail and waiting for help is most often the best option for adults and always the best option for children.

- **BE ESPECIALLY CAREFUL WHEN CROSSING STREAMS.** Whether you are fording the stream or crossing on a log, make every step count. If you have any doubt about maintaining your balance on a foot log, go ahead and ford the stream instead. When fording a stream, use a trekking pole or stout stick for balance and face upstream as you cross. If a stream seems too deep to ford, turn back. Whatever is on the other side is not worth risking your life.

- **BE CAREFUL AT OVERLOOKS.** While these areas may provide spectacular views, they are potentially hazardous. Stay back from the edge of outcrops and be absolutely sure of your footing; a misstep can mean a nasty and possibly fatal fall.

- **KNOW THE SYMPTOMS OF HYPOTHERMIA.** Shivering and forgetfulness are the two most common indicators of this insidious killer. Hypothermia can occur at any elevation, even in the summer, especially when the hiker is wearing lightweight cotton clothing. If symptoms arise, get the victim shelter, hot liquids, and dry clothes or a dry sleeping bag.

- **TAKE ALONG YOUR BRAIN.** A cool, calculating mind is the single most important piece of equipment you'll ever need on the trail. Think before you act. Watch your step. Plan ahead. Avoiding accidents before they happen is the best recipe for a rewarding and relaxing hike.

KIM'S TIPS FOR CAMPING WITH KIDS . . .

Camping with children can be a great way to introduce the young to the outdoors. It's also wonderful exercise and an even better family-bonding experience. It's time away from laundry, cell phones, and school—just you and the kids and nature.

WHAT TO BRING Packing for the kids is much like packing for the parents. Be sure each camper has the USDA Forest Service's "ten essentials": map, compass, water, knife, waterproof matches, high-energy food, suitable extra clothing (such as rain gear), mirror, first-aid kit, and whistle.

Consider packing my list of additional "ten kid essentials" for the tent: your child's favorite wholesome snack, juice, sunglasses, sunscreen, baby wipes, kid's trail map, kid's magnifying glass, scavenger-hunt cards, cuddle buddy, and permanent markers.

Be sure everyone is dressed for the weather. For hot or cold days, the rule is to dress in layers. All children need to have one proper pair of socks and one proper pair of shoes. Be sure there is no cotton in the socks, since cotton retains moisture and helps create blisters. Instead, buy child-sized wool socks and nylon liners—there are many different weights and variations for any condition.

Each child needs a sleeping bag that will fit his or her body type and provide warmth at night. Do your research on sizes and temperature ratings. (Don't cave in and get the Barbie sleeping bag little Susie *really* wants. Save that for slumber parties indoors.)

SAFETY CONSIDERATIONS Children should be taught from the get-go that they must stay within eyesight of an adult. They are to never run off. Not only can they get lost or injured, they can cause damage to the ecosystem. Teach your kids to treat the outdoors kindly, and the outdoors will repay the favor. Also teach children to stay where they are if they get lost. Many children relate to hugging a tree when lost—instruct them to find one, hold on, and blow their whistle. Three whistle blows is the standard distress signal, which indicates, "I am lost" or "I need help." Never let kids go near steep cliffs and other drop-off areas. Rules about rivers and other water sources and climbing on accessible rocks must be addressed as well. (My rule is "No!")

Always teach outdoor etiquette: Leave no trace, pick up after others who do not, and don't pick or pull anything. And of course, leaves of three, let them be.

KEEP IT FUN Before you leave home, have the kids help make a special kid-friendly map of the campground area that they can keep in their bag. Making maps helps teach direction and creativity. Create a kid-friendly legend that has items like waterfalls, trails, trees, or tents. Have the child mark interesting points of interest while they are camping.

Toy stores are home to many camping or backyard camping things such as kids' magnifying glasses. A magnifying glass can be used to identify plants, insects, minerals in rocks, and flowers.

Make scavenger-hunt cards to use on any hike away from the campground (or in the area around the campground). A stack of index cards works fine. Have your child cut camping-related items from used magazines and paste them on each card. If your child can draw, this works as well. Write the name under the item and bring as many as you want. You can prolong your scavenger hunt cards throughout the summer by simply marking each item that you see on the back. It's fun to have a trump card that could be tucked away for special sightings: bull snake, lost watch, or an abandoned sock. Bring a permanent marker to take notes on your cards—some may even want to laminate their cards.

Play games like "I Spy," try bird-watching, look for animal tracks, or simply count rocks in the campground. The key is to play games that encourage children to observe their surroundings.

Assign a camping leader (or mountain leader as we call it) and have that child guide the camping trip. Have them plan the menu, decide when meals will be served, and even let them pick bedtime (don't worry; most campers go to bed when the sun goes down). Have your child invite a friend, which helps your child see the world from another youngster's perspective.

If the camping trip is going well, be sure to head home a little early; it prevents a last-minute meltdown. It's always better to end early on a positive note than to end with sore feet, a lot of whining, and discouraged hikers.

... AND CAMPING WITH DOGS

I love camping with my dog as long as she doesn't bark at strange noises in the middle of the night. Use these basic guidelines when taking your hound into the wild.

- Leash a dog to prevent it from chasing wildlife and other campground users.

- Also leash a dog to keep it from drinking out of streams and other water sources. Harmful bacteria, such as giardia, are a threat to dogs as well as humans. Always pack water for your dog.

- Further, leash a dog to keep it from getting lost and possibly attacked by wild animals. Few things are worse than having to take a dog to the vet on a weekend with porcupine quills lodged in its sinuses.

- Make sure that all of your dog's vaccinations and medications are current, including rabies, bordetella, and heartworm. If you're planning to camp in an area with Lyme disease, ask your vet about vaccinations.

- After camping, carefully check Fido for ticks and burrs. Prepare for accidents, and keep antibiotic cream and self-sticking bandage tape in your first-aid kid.

- It's essential to pack out dog poop rather than leave it at the campsite. Dog waste is not the same as that of other animals, even that of coyotes or wolves. It's dangerous to the environment, especially near water sources, and it makes a bad impression on the campers who use the site after you.

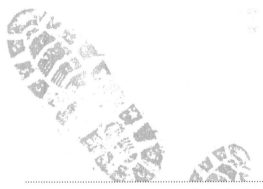

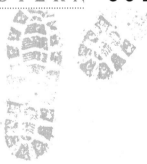

EASTERN COLORADO

1
BONNY LAKE STATE PARK CAMPGROUND

BONNY LAKE IS THE MOST EASTERLY campground in this entire guidebook. Located in a wide valley of the South Fork of the Republican River near the Kansas border, this 1,900-acre reservoir was originally built by the U.S. Bureau of Reclamation in the 1950s. The state of Colorado transformed it into a state park in the 1970s. Now you can boat, swim, and fish in this surprisingly scenic slice of the prairie. The East Beach is the best in tent camping among a good group of campgrounds that circle the lake. If you are coming from out of state, stop here on your way to or from the mountains. You will realize that Colorado really is beautiful not only in the high country, but in the prairie as well.

Starting on the northwest side of Bonny Lake is Foster Grove Campground. Cottonwood and willow shade the grassy flat of the campsites, though there is very little undergrowth and thus very little campsite privacy. However, the campsites are spread apart, making lack of privacy less of an issue. The lake is visible, but it is about a half-mile distant. Foster Grove is the second most developed campground here. It has showers and flush toilets.

North Cove is on a small arm of the lake. The campground is smaller, but more popular than Foster Grove. Ten of the 21 campsites face the lake. The sites away from the lake have metal shade shelters over the picnic tables. Although there is no electricity, bigger rigs still dominate this campground. There are vault toilets and water spigots, too. A boat ramp and small dock is at one end of the campground with a horseshoe pit nearby.

The East Beach Campground is at the southeastern corner of the reservoir near the dam. Drive in and pass three sunny campsites near the lake—they are screened from a view of the beach area by a line of

> *Bonny Lake is your prairie getaway in northeastern Colorado.*

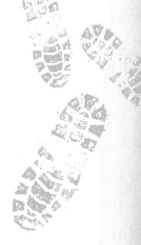

RATINGS

Beauty: ✿ ✿ ✿ ✿
Privacy: ✿ ✿ ✿
Spaciousness: ✿ ✿ ✿
Quiet: ✿ ✿ ✿ ✿
Security: ✿ ✿ ✿ ✿
Cleanliness: ✿ ✿ ✿ ✿ ✿

ADDRESS: Bonny Lake State Park
30010 County Road 3
Idalia, CO 80735

OPERATED BY: Colorado State Parks

INFORMATION: (970) 354-7306;
parks.state.co.us;
Bonny marina and
store, (970) 354-7339

OPEN: All year

SITES: 10 walk-in tent sites,
190 other

EACH SITE HAS: Walk-in tent sites
have picnic table
and stand-up grill;
others also have
electricity

ASSIGNMENT: By advance reservation or pick an avail-
able site on arrival

REGISTRATION: By phone (call (800)
678-CAMP or (303)
470-1144 in Denver)
or at www.reserve
america.com

FACILITIES: Coin-operated hot
showers, flush and
vault toilets, laun-
dry, phone, vending
machines, group
picnic area, marina

PARKING: At campsites or
walk-in tent campers
parking area

FEE: $5 Parks Pass plus
$12 North Cove, East
Beach; $12 Foster
Grove, $12–$16
electric sites. Add $8
reservation fee.

ELEVATION: 3,700 feet

RESTRICTIONS: *Pets:* On leash only
Fires: In fire grates
only
Alcohol: 3.2% beer
only
Vehicles: Designated
roads only
Other: 14-day stay
limit in 30-day period

cottonwoods. Under this line of cottonwoods are the park's best campsites. This is a row of ten walk-in tent sites, which are by the lake under the trees and have a view of the beautiful waters. Try to get these campsites. Farther on are 20 more campsites exposed to the extremes of the prairie; mainly open exposure, high winds, and blazing sunshine. Thankfully, they do have shade shelters. The lake dam stands tall to your right.

On the southern shore of Bonny Lake near the main body of park development is Wagon Wheel Campground. It has all the amenities including laundry facilities, a dump station, and electricity—this means RVs. Stay away from this campground. A boat launch and marina are nearby.

This is but one of three boat launches scattered around this reservoir with the blue waters. Waterskiing is very popular here, but skiers must make their wakes in designated areas only. You can rent small fishing boats and pontoons at the marina here, and if you already have a boat, storage facilities are available as well. Limited supplies are available here, but I suggest loading up in Burlington.

Bonny Lake is known as one of the best warmwater fisheries in Colorado. Wipers, walleye, pike, bass, and bluegill can be caught in season. Call ahead to the state park for the latest fishing report. Beach lovers don't have to leave land-locked Colorado to get a little sand between their toes. Bonny Lake has several beach areas. West Beach is one of the designated swimming areas. The other designated swimming beach is near the marina. Other beach areas are not designated for swimming.

Bring a bike and pedal around the lake. The view of the waters and the prairie from the dam is vivid. Bonny Lake is not just for summer. Wildlife viewing is a year-round pastime here. Bird life is particularly abundant. Hunting is allowed in season. No matter what time of year, you will be pleasantly surprised at Bonny Lake.

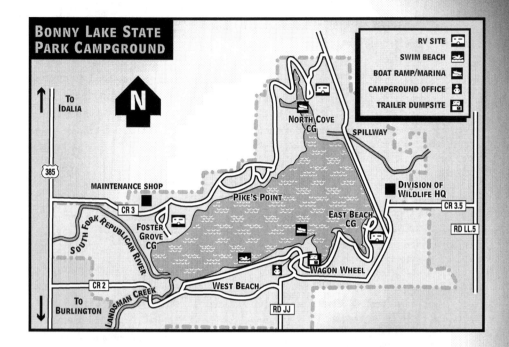

BONNY LAKE STATE PARK CAMPGROUND

Legend:
- RV SITE
- SWIM BEACH
- BOAT RAMP/MARINA
- CAMPGROUND OFFICE
- TRAILER DUMPSITE

To IDALIA

N

385

NORTH COVE CG

SPILLWAY

MAINTENANCE SHOP

PIKE'S POINT

DIVISION OF WILDLIFE HQ

CR 3

CR 3.5

SOUTH FORK REPUBLICAN RIVER

FOSTER GROVE CG

EAST BEACH CG

RD LL.5

CR 2

LANDSMAN CREEK

WEST BEACH

WAGON WHEEL

To BURLINGTON

RD JJ

GETTING THERE

From I-70 in Burlington, drive north on US 385 for 23 miles to CR 2. Turn right on CR 2 and follow it 1.5 miles to Bonny Lake State Park.

GPS COORDINATES

UTM Zone (WGS84) 13S
Easting 0741440
Northing 4388090
Latitude N 39° 36' 30.8"
Longitude W 102° 11' 16"

> *Enjoy shoreline camping on this high-plains reservoir.*

JACKSON LAKE, A LARGE, WARM-WATER reservoir, is an important feature of the northeastern Colorado high plains landscape. Local farmers depend on its water to irrigate their lands. But before these waters grace the fields, they provide scenic recreational opportunities to all who are lucky enough to come this way. The Rocky Mountains will always be a draw, but this relaxing state park should not be overlooked. Campers can stay overnight in a slew of shoreline campsites while boating, sailing, swimming, and fishing on the 2,700-acre lake. A walk-in tent camping area and lakeside beaches make this oasis even more appealing.

Several campgrounds border the impoundment along the west shore. The Lakeside Campground has wide-open, sun-whipped campsites farther from the lake, but nearer to the water, cottonwoods shade the preferred lakeside sites. A camper services building and shadier campsites are closer to the lake. Then a set of walk-in tent sites stretches along the shoreline. These are the best sites in the park for tent campers. A beach swimming area is near these walk-in tent sites.

The Cove Campground is more open. It has electrical hookups and caters more to RVs. The campsite picnic tables are shaded with interesting shelters that look like the shell of a turtle turned sideways. There is access to the swim beach here as well. The Pelican Campground also has four walk-in tent sites a slight distance from the shore and some shady shoreline drive-up campsites. Many of the others are more exposed to the elements. Boaters will want to take advantage of the quick access to the Shore-line Marina and boat ramp just north of the Pelican Campground.

The next campground, Sandpiper, lies on an open slope with numerous planted trees. The height of the hill allows for a great view of the lake, but at the

RATINGS

Beauty: ✿ ✿ ✿
Privacy: ✿ ✿ ✿
Spaciousness: ✿ ✿ ✿ ✿ ✿
Quiet: ✿ ✿ ✿
Security: ✿ ✿ ✿ ✿ ✿
Cleanliness: ✿ ✿ ✿ ✿ ✿

expense of shade and privacy. There is a camper's services building and electrical hookups here. Fox Hills is on a wide slope that offers views of the prairie and lake, which is fairly distant. There are many trees here. The final campground on the west shore, Northview, is on an open slope, but has electrical hookups and shade shelters for the campsite picnic tables. These last three campgrounds should be your last choice.

There is one small campground, Dunes, on the south shore of Jackson Lake. This campground abuts some wooded dunes that separate you from the lake, but the water is just a short climb over the dunes. The campground has picnic shelters, but also Russian olive and cottonwood trees for shade. These are more popular sites, and the small size of this campground makes for a quiet camping experience.

Water sports dominate the activities at Jackson Lake. Jet skiing, power boating, and waterskiing are enjoyed during summer months. The Shoreline Marina has limited supplies and most anything a boater might need, including boats themselves, from jet skis to pontoon barges. The west and south shores are designated as wakeless areas. In these areas are two lakeside beaches where swimmers cool off in the waters and sunbathers soak up some rays on the sand.

Bank fishing is popular in the Dike Fishing Area, where boats are prohibited. Both warm- and cold-water species inhabit the reservoir. Trout, walleye, wiper, perch, and crappie are angled for from the Dike Fishing Area and throughout the lake on boats. Anglers who go ice fishing on Jackson Lake increase each winter.

Landlubbers will be seen bicycling on the park roads. Campers can enjoy interpretive programs on summer weekends. You may learn about Jackson Lake's wildlife, especially the wealth of waterfowl. Whether on land or water, you will come away from this pride of the prairie with a new perspective on Colorado.

KEY INFORMATION

ADDRESS:	Jackson Lake State Park 26363 CR 3 Orchard, CO 80649
OPERATED BY:	Colorado State Parks
INFORMATION:	(970) 645-2551; parks.state.co.us
OPEN:	All year
SITES:	262
EACH SITE HAS:	Picnic table, fire ring
ASSIGNMENT:	By reservation or pick an available site upon arrival
REGISTRATION:	(800) 678-CAMP (2267) or (303) 470-1144 in Denver), at entrance station or park office, or online at www .reserveamerica .com
FACILITIES:	Hot showers, flush and vault toilets, laundry facilities, phone, electricity, marina
PARKING:	At campsites or walk-in tent campers parking area
FEE:	$5 Parks Pass plus, $12 basic sites, $16 electric sites. An $8 reservation fee is additional.
ELEVATION:	4,440 feet
RESTRICTIONS:	*Pets:* On leash only *Fires:* In fire grates only *Alcohol:* 3.2% beer only *Vehicles:* None *Other:* 14-day stay limit in a 30-day period

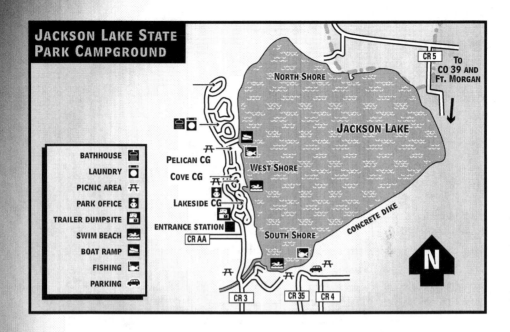

GETTING THERE

From Fort Morgan, head west on I-76 for 14 miles to exit 66 and CO 39. Head north on CO 39 and follow it for 7.3 miles to CR Y5. Turn left on CR Y5 and follow it 2.5 miles to Jackson Lake State Park.

GPS COORDINATES

UTM Zone (WGS84)   13T
Easting   0577140
Northing   4470680
Latitude   N 40° 22' 50.1"
Longitude   W 104° 5' 24"

3
PAWNEE NATIONAL GRASSLAND CAMPGROUND

I**F THE COLORADO MOUNTAINS** are what make the state famous, then the Colorado prairies are the lesser-known better half. And the humble prairie folk are okay with that. The uninterrupted vistas and heritage of Northeastern Colorado is an open book of nature with its own distinct and fragile beauty. Less populated and less trampled by tourists, this area is prime for discovery. Tent campgrounds are extremely limited east of I-25; the main interstate artery that loosely splits the state in half and serves as a vein to the Colorado Front Range. So, we are pleased to point you in the direction of Pawnee National Grassland and the Crow Valley Recreation Area.

Traveling across the Pawnee Pioneer Trail Scenic and Historic Byway, you may imagine how this short grass prairie was viewed by Native Americans, frontier men and women, early cattle ranchers, homesteaders, and those who faced the Dust Bowl and Great Depression of the 1930s. After the failure of many farms during this last timeframe, the US government purchased land from bankrupt farmers and instituted methods to restore the land and vegetation damaged by years of drought, plowing, wind, and water; thus creating the Pawnee National Grassland. Today, the Pawnee National Grassland covers almost 200,000 acres mixed with private land and is an internationally known birding area. Hiking, camping, picnicking, mountain biking, and sight-seeing are also popular recreational activities.

The campground is just past the entrance to the Crow Valley Recreation Area, which is only a quarter-mile off of CR 77. When you enter, pass by group picnicking and camping sites and the turn off for the education site. The Crow Valley Campground sits along Crow Creek and the entrance is right next to the Birdwalk trailhead. A grove of elm and cottonwood

> *Head east for a high-plains pioneer experience.*

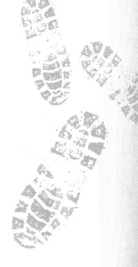

RATINGS

Beauty: ☆ ☆ ☆ ☆
Privacy: ☆ ☆ ☆ ☆
Spaciousness: ☆ ☆ ☆
Quiet: ☆ ☆ ☆ ☆
Security: ☆ ☆ ☆
Cleanliness: ☆ ☆ ☆

ADDRESS:	Pawnee National Grassland 660 "O" Street Greeley, CO 80631
OPERATED BY:	USDA Forest Service, Arapaho and Roosevelt National Forests, Pawnee National Grassland
INFORMATION:	(970) 346-5000, www.fs.fed.us.r2/arnf
OPEN:	Mid-February–mid-December
SITES:	10
EACH SITE HAS:	Picnic table, fire pit
ASSIGNMENT:	First come, first served
REGISTRATION:	On site
FACILITIES:	Water, vault toilets, horseshoe pits, volleyball court, baseball field, and farm museum
PARKING:	At campsite
FEE:	$10 for a single unit, $14 for a double unit
ELEVATION:	4,856 feet
RESTRICTIONS:	*Pets:* On leash *Fires:* In designated fire pits *Alcohol:* Allowed *Vehicles:* 35 feet *Other:* 14-day stay limit; single units hold 5 people, double units hold 10 people

trees provides a unique respite in an otherwise open prairie. There are ten individual sites and they begin in a counterclockwise layout around a perfect circle. All campsites meet ADA requirements for handicap accessibility. (There are also two accessible trails in the campground.) One double unit is available for those with special needs and the rangers ask that you leave this unit open until all other spaces are filled. Sites 1, 2, and 3 are single campsites on the outer edge of the circle. Following them are sites 4, 5, and 6 which are the three double campsites. Sites 7, 8, 9, and 10 are closer to Crow Creek and sit on the western edge of the circle. Site 9 is the only site in the middle of the circle.

May and June are the best months to come because the bird migration is in full swing, wildflowers are in bloom, and it is much cooler than the blazing July and August months. Even during the cooler months, finding a shady campsite among the ten is paramount. Large cottonwood trees shade the sites that ring the outer fringe of the campground. From these sites are short trails that lead through the Crow Valley cottonwood groves and river thickets that attract birds and birders in large numbers. July and August are not only hot, but the mosquitoes swarm. If you come during these hot months be prepared.

Pawnee National Grassland offers hiking opportunities directly from the campground and within the prairie. The Pawnee Buttes are 30 miles northeast of the Crow Valley Recreation Area. The Buttes rise 300 feet above the surrounding prairie and they are the result of erosion of uplifted sedimentary beds deposited by ancient seas. The trail is open all year and it is an easy 1.5-mile hike to the base of the western Pawnee Butte.

Pawnee National Grassland supports many bird species, especially during migration. The Colorado state bird, the lark bunting, is very common in the prairie in the spring and summer. A pamphlet, describing a self-guided motor vehicle bird tour of the west side of the Pawnee National Grassland and is available in Crow Valley. A brochure entitled "Birding on the Pawnee by Automobile or Mountain Bike" is even available for mountain bikers. The history of the area

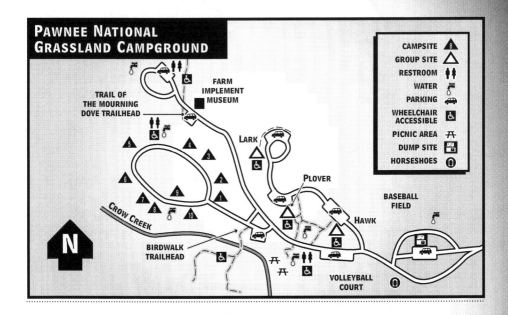

PAWNEE NATIONAL GRASSLAND CAMPGROUND

CAMPSITE	▲
GROUP SITE	△
RESTROOM	�
WATER	≡
PARKING	🚗
WHEELCHAIR ACCESSIBLE	♿
PICNIC AREA	⊼
DUMP SITE	▣
HORSESHOES	◉

TRAIL OF THE MOURNING DOVE TRAILHEAD

FARM IMPLEMENT MUSEUM

LARK

PLOVER

BASEBALL FIELD

HAWK

CROW CREEK

BIRDWALK TRAILHEAD

VOLLEYBALL COURT

is represented by many cemeteries and small museums and preserved homesteads. Artifacts, arrowheads, fossils, and antique barnwood are easy to spot, but you must leave these items untouched.

Keep this campground at the top of your flatland list. It is an eye-opening experience to witness the magic of Colorado from the solitude of its open spaces. The mountain views are much different here than anywhere else in the state with distant views of the snow-capped peaks. Large, fluffy clouds turn into dark thunderheads in a snap and lightning illuminates the beasts, creating quite a show. This, along with the promise of no crowds and your pick of campsites, should seal the deal.

GETTING THERE

From the intersection of I-25 and CO 14, take CO 14 east 37 miles to Weld County Road CR 77. Take CR 77 a quarter-mile to the campground.

GPS COORDINATES

UTM Zone (WGS84)   13T
Easting   0556020
Northing   4499450
Latitude   N 40 °38' 45"
Longitude   W 104° 20' 14"

THE BEST IN TENT CAMPING COLORADO

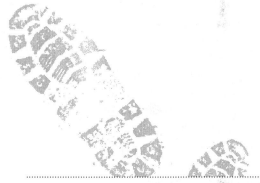

NORTH CENTRAL **COLORADO**

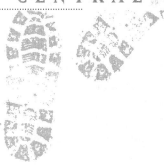

4
BROWNS PARK
CAMPGROUND

THE LOWER **L**ARAMIE **R**IVER **VALLEY** has a big-country-lonesome feel to it. There aren't too many folks around here, mainly just ranchers. Browns Park is tucked away in some woods on a side creek that feeds into the Laramie. If you want to get away from the people that are trying to get away Browns Park is tucked away in some woods on a side creek that feeds into the laramie. If you want to get away from the people who are trying to get away from it all, come here. This pretty little campground is adjacent to the woods and lakes of the Rawah Wilderness, which covers a stretch of the Medicine Bow Mountains. You can hike and fish here, or just take it easy. Browns Park is great for relaxation. Summer afternoons are as slow as molasses.

After passing the busy campgrounds of the Poudre Canyon and overcrowded Chambers Lake, you'll feel grateful for the peace and quiet here in the Laramie Valley.

A couple of sites lie in the lodgepole and aspen woods to your right, then the main campground drive splits off to the right and you enter the outer loop. (There used to be one more split off to the right, but the beavers took care of that.) The outer loop turns away from Jinks Creek and runs alongside a slight slope.

The campsites on the outside of the loop are higher than the road, but have been graded and host tent pads for a level night of rest. The inner loop campsites lie in a mixed wood with a very grassy understory augmented by small conifers. Move away from the hill and pass the inner loop. These campsites are more open, but all of the campsites are spread far apart, so privacy can be had by every camper. The inner loop splits Browns Park in half, but the roads are spread far enough apart that you won't be bothered by your fellow campers when they drive past. The county

> *Browns Park abuts the old-growth forests and alpine lakes of the Rawah Wilderness near the Wyoming border.*

RATINGS

Beauty: ✿ ✿ ✿ ✿
Privacy: ✿ ✿ ✿
Spaciousness: ✿ ✿ ✿ ✿
Quiet: ✿ ✿ ✿ ✿
Security: ✿ ✿ ✿
Cleanliness: ✿ ✿ ✿

ADDRESS: Browns Park
Campground
Canyon Lakes
Ranger District
2150 Centre Avenue,
Builing E
Fort Collins, CO
80526

OPERATED BY: USDA Forest Service, Arapaho and
Roosevelt National
Forests, Pawnee
National Grassland

INFORMATION: (970) 295-6700;
www.fs.fed.us/r2/
arnf

OPEN: May–September

SITES: 28

EACH SITE HAS: Tent pad, picnic
table, fire grate,
stand-up grill

ASSIGNMENT: First come,
first served; no
reservations

REGISTRATION: Self-registration on
site

FACILITIES: Vault toilet
(no water)

PARKING: At campsites only

FEE: $11 per night

ELEVATION: 8,400 feet

RESTRICTIONS: *Pets:* On leash only
Fires: In fire grates
only
Alcohol: At campsites
only
Vehicles: 30 feet
Other: 14-day stay
limit

road leading in to Browns Park gets less traffic than some campgrounds I've seen.

Complete your loop back to the campground entrance and the new vault toilets. Browns Park has no water—I recommend bringing it with you.

This site has low usage. I met a man on my visit who had been coming to Browns Park for ten years and had only seen the campground full once. He and his wife were the only campers there on the day I met him. Weekdays can be desolate, which is great for those who love solitude. Summer weekends can be half to two-thirds full, except when the campground fills up for major holidays.

For a nearby natural experience, check out the beaver pond and see if you find any of nature's architects plotting to flood the rest of the campground. Two hiking trails leave from the trailhead adjacent to Browns Park into the Rawah Wilderness, which is far enough from the metropolitan areas to receive little use also.

The McIntyre Trail traces McIntyre Creek to Houseman Park, and then turns left to another meadow where beavers have again been busy flooding the trail. These upper beaver ponds offer excellent trout fishing. The Link Trail climbs through a lodgepole forest to a former burned area, where views of the Laramie River valley stretch into Wyoming. You can also see the Poudre Canyon below.

If you want to access the high lakes of the Medicine Bows, take the Rawah Trail, which starts in the Laramie River valley south of Browns Park (you pass this trailhead on the way in). The Rawah Trail crosses several different environments. Leave the valley grasslands, wind your way from lodgepole to spruce–fir forest to tundra above the tree line, where there are many bodies of water collectively dubbed the Rawah Lakes.

No matter what you do, bring some friends with you to Browns Park and the Medicine Bows because there might not be too many other people out here, especially during the week. Also, bring all the supplies you may need because the nearest store is not really near at all, though there is a guest ranch nearby down Larimer CR 103.

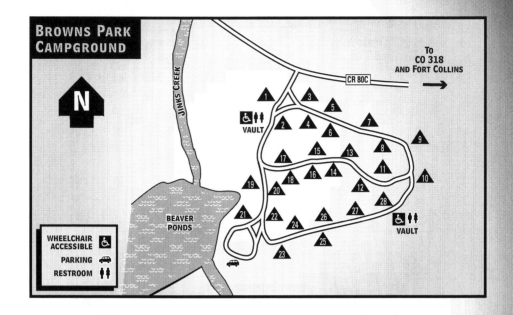

GETTING THERE

From Fort Collins drive north on US 287 for 11 miles to CO 14. Turn left on CO 14 and follow it for 49 miles west to CR 103 (Laramie River Road). Turn right on CR 103 and follow it for 15 miles. At a T-intersection turn left on CR 80C and travel approximately 3 miles to Browns Park campground.

GPS COORDINATES

UTM Zone (WGS84)	13T
Easting	0421780
Northing	4516650
Latitude	N 40° 47' 49.7"
Longitude	W 105° 55' 37"

5
BUFFALO
CAMPGROUND

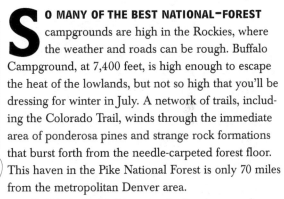

> *Buffalo is a quick getaway for metro Denver–area mountain bikers, hikers, and families.*

SO MANY OF THE BEST NATIONAL-FOREST campgrounds are high in the Rockies, where the weather and roads can be rough. Buffalo Campground, at 7,400 feet, is high enough to escape the heat of the lowlands, but not so high that you'll be dressing for winter in July. A network of trails, including the Colorado Trail, winds through the immediate area of ponderosa pines and strange rock formations that burst forth from the needle-carpeted forest floor. This haven in the Pike National Forest is only 70 miles from the metropolitan Denver area.

Buffalo is situated in a stand of mature ponderosa pine on a gentle slope. Flowers, grasses, and juniper ground cover spread over the open, parklike forest floor. An ideal mix of sun and shade makes its way through the evergreens onto the very large campsites. The largest of tents will have no problem setting up on leveled areas at each campsite. But this openness cuts down on camper privacy.

Pass the fee station and begin climbing up the hillside. Pass an inner loop that splits off to your left and has seven campsites that are more open than most because they border a small clearing in the center of the main loop. Most of the campsites are on the outside of the main loop and extend far back from the road. The higher you are on the loop, the better you can see a stone outcrop across the way where rock climbers go to work.

A campground host is stationed on the loop to quell any late-night parties or direct you to many of the recreation opportunities in the area. The campground was recently refurbished, and its vault toilets have been replaced. The three water spigots are very reliable.

You can reserve a site here, but Buffalo rarely fills, barring major summer holidays. Weekends usually see

RATINGS

Beauty: ✩ ✩ ✩ ✩
Privacy: ✩ ✩
Spaciousness: ✩ ✩ ✩ ✩ ✩
Quiet: ✩ ✩ ✩
Security: ✩ ✩ ✩ ✩
Cleanliness: ✩ ✩ ✩

a mix of families and youthful active folks, the vast majority of whom are tent campers. Buffalo is quiet during the week; you can be assured of a campsite. No matter when you come, there is plenty to enjoy in the surrounding Pike National Forest.

As mentioned, rock climbers scale the formation across from the campground. Mountain bikers are seen everywhere, riding the trails that wind through the Buffalo Recreation Area and beyond. A favorite ride is the Colorado Trail. Keep going up the hill from the campground and you will intersect the trail. You can turn left out of the campground on the Colorado Trail and bike to CO 126, then return via FS 550. Trail 722 makes a loop off the Colorado Trail south. Just off FS 550, there is another loop that heads toward Miller Gulch. Make up your own loop in the trails that twist and turn amid the pines and pillars of stone.

Buffalo Creek, flowing just below the campground, offers trout fishing and more mountain biking along FS 543 that parallels Buffalo. Still more biking trails splinter off FS 543. Wellington Lake, at the upper drainage of Buffalo Creek, is a private lake that offers boat rentals and trout fishing for a fee.

Hikers can enjoy the same trails as the mountain bikers, but at a slower speed. You can also head into the Lost Creek Wilderness, just a few miles northwest of Buffalo. From the trailhead off Wellington Lake Road, hikers can take the Colorado Trail into the wilderness high country or walk the Craig Meadows Trail into Craig Creek. Other hikes into this wilderness are also accessible from this trailhead.

In the summer there is still enough light to make the drive from Denver or Colorado Springs and be sitting at Buffalo at dusk by the campfire, where you can cook up a good supper, then retire to your tent. Next morning you can jump out of the tent and onto your favorite trail.

ADDRESS: Buffalo Campground South Platte Ranger District 19316 Goddard Ranch Court Morrison, CO 80465

OPERATED BY: USDA Forest Service, Pike and San Isabel National Forests, Cimarron and Comanche National Grasslands

INFORMATION: (303) 275-5610; www.fs.fed.us/r2/psicc/spl

OPEN: Mid-May– Labor Day

SITES: 41

EACH SITE HAS: Picnic table, fire ring, tent pad

ASSIGNMENT: By reservation or first come, first served if site available

REGISTRATION: Call (877) 444-6777), visit www.reserveusa.com, or self-register on site

FACILITIES: Water spigot, vault toilet

PARKING: At campsites only

FEE: $12 per night, an additional $9 fee added to each Internet or phone reservation

ELEVATION: 7,400 feet

RESTRICTIONS: *Pets:* On leash only
Fires: In fire rings only
Alcohol: At campsites only
Vehicles: 22 feet
Other: 14-day stay limit

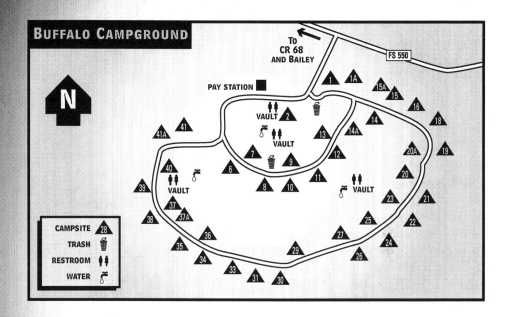

GETTING THERE

From US 285 in Bailey, head southeast on CR 68 (it turns into FS 543) for 8 miles to FS 550. Turn left on FS 550 (Redskin Creek Road) and follow it 4 miles to Buffalo (not Buffalo Springs) Campground, which will be on your right.

GPS COORDINATES

UTM Zone (WGS84)   13S
Easting   0471140
Northing   4354840
Latitude   N 39° 20' 32.9"
Longitude   W 105° 20' 8.3"

6
BYERS CREEK CAMPGROUND

GRAND **C**OUNTY **PRIDES ITSELF** as the mountain-biking capital of Colorado. And maybe it is. More than 600 miles of single track, old logging roads, and fire roads are ready for avid pedalers. The Fraser Valley gently slopes up to the rugged Rockies, allowing for varied slopes to suit a bicycler's varied desires. Many of the trails have been improved to attract mountain bikers. Nearby ski resorts, including Sol Vista, Silver Creek, Winter Park, and Mary Jane offer lifts, making rides a little faster. Not only bikers, but hikers and anglers also need a good tent-camping locale. This beautiful valley, rimmed by granite peaks and Byers Creek, is it.

The campground lies in the Saint Louis Valley between the Byers Peak Wilderness and the Vasquez Peak Wilderness. At the head of the valley is Saint Louis Peak; the Fraser Valley is below. The air cools a bit while driving into the Fraser Experimental Forest where Byers Creek Campground is located. Turn into the campground and note the density of the woods here. Lodgepoles are crowded together with spruce and other conifers, especially along the creek. The thick understory indicates less use than most campgrounds.

Also note the cleanliness of the campground and its overall well-kept appearance. Byers Creek is operated jointly by the USDA Forest Service and a local Lions Club—and a good job is done by all. The first campsite is on your left just before the small loop begins. The next few campsites on the loop are down from the road in a flat along Saint Louis Creek. These sites are for water lovers. Byers Creek flows in upstream and across from the road.

As the road curves left, the only broken stretch of forest is in a flood plain to your right.

A few more campsites sit on a rise away from Byers Creek, but the sites themselves have been leveled.

> *Byers Creek is mountain-biking headquarters for the Fraser Valley. There are also two wilderness areas nearby.*

RATINGS

Beauty: ✿ ✿ ✿ ✿
Privacy: ✿ ✿ ✿
Spaciousness: ✿ ✿ ✿ ✿
Quiet: ✿ ✿ ✿ ✿
Security: ✿ ✿ ✿
Cleanliness: ✿ ✿ ✿ ✿

ADDRESS: Byers Creek
Campground
Sulphur Ranger
District
9 Ten Mile Drive,
P.O. Box 10
Granby, CO
80446-0010

OPERATED BY: USDA Forest Service, Arapaho and
Roosevelt National
Forests, Pawnee
National Grassland

INFORMATION: (970) 887-4100;
www.fs.fed.us/r2/
arnf

OPEN: Memorial Day–
Labor Day

SITES: 6

EACH SITE HAS: Picnic table, fire ring

ASSIGNMENT: First come, first
served; no
reservation

REGISTRATION: Self-registration on
site

FACILITIES: Hand pump well,
vault toilets

PARKING: At campsites only

FEE: $12 per night

ELEVATION: 9,360 feet

RESTRICTIONS: *Pets:* On leash only
Fires: In fire grates
only
Alcohol: At campsites
only
Vehicles: 32 feet
Other: 14-day stay
limit

The water and rest rooms are in the center of the loop. This is one pretty, intimate campground. But its small size means fewer sites, and that means the possibility of it being full when you arrive. You needn't worry during the week. It usually will fill on weekends because it is not difficult to fill a six-site campground. (An alternative is the Saint Louis Creek campground 3 miles northeast of Byers Creek. It is not the best in tent camping, but it will do in a pinch.)

Before you drive up to Byers Creek, stop in the Fraser Visitor Center. It is located near the first turn toward the campground. It has some excellent information about biking in the area, including a full-color mountain bike trail map of Winter Park and the Fraser Valley. The map shows miles of trails and rates them by difficulty. There is even a bike trail leaving from the Visitor Center itself.

The trails include forest roads that you can take right from the campground. The west side of Grand County has lesser-used trails. The majority of trails are on public land, so you can concentrate on pedaling instead of worrying whether you are trespassing. Anyway, local folks embrace mountain bikers. From June through September, mountain biking events are held here, including races and festivals.

The Fraser Valley is not only about mountain biking, however. It is also about hiking and fishing. Half of the 8,095-acre Byers Peak Wilderness is tundra. Wilderness areas do not allow bikes, but you can hike the trail to the top of Byers Peak. The trailhead is 3 miles from the campground, and then it's a 3-mile round-trip to the top of the 12,804-foot mountain. Much of the nearby Vasquez Peak Wilderness is above the tree line too. Forest roads splinter off Saint Louis Road, offering hikes into the high country of both wildernesses.

At the head of Saint Louis Road is the 3-mile trail to Saint Louis Lake. You can also reach Saint Louis Peak from here. Anglers can fish the 11,500-foot Saint Louis Lake. There are 8 miles of fishing on Saint Louis Creek as well. I've only touched on a few of the many outdoor opportunities here.

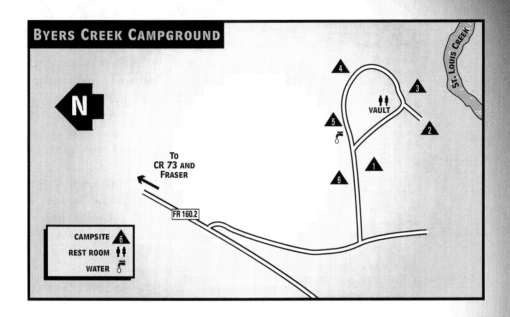

BYERS CREEK CAMPGROUND

N

To
CR 73 AND
FRASER

VAULT

FR 160.2

CAMPSITE	6
REST ROOM	♀♂
WATER	⌀

St. Louis Creek

Make Byers Creek your tent-camping headquarters for the Fraser Valley, then proceed with your favorite activity.

GETTING THERE

From Fraser, head west on CR 72 (Elk Creek Road). Follow CR 72 for 0.4 mile to Fraser Parkway (a dirt road). Turn right on Fraser Parkway and follow it for 0.7 mile to CR 73 (Saint Louis Creek Road). Turn left on CR 73 and follow it for 7 miles to Byers Creek Campground, which will be on your left.

GPS COORDINATES

UTM Zone (WGS84)	13S
Easting	0422990
Northing	4414250
Latitude	N 39° 52' 30.5"
Longitude	W 105° 54' 0.6"

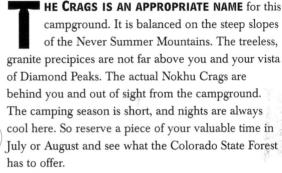

THE CRAGS CAMPGROUND

> *Colorado State Forest is rich in wildlife and is one of the state's best places to see moose.*

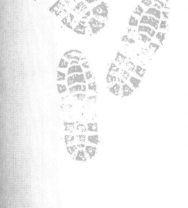

THE **CRAGS IS AN APPROPRIATE NAME** for this campground. It is balanced on the steep slopes of the Never Summer Mountains. The treeless, granite precipices are not far above you and your vista of Diamond Peaks. The actual Nokhu Crags are behind you and out of sight from the campground. The camping season is short, and nights are always cool here. So reserve a piece of your valuable time in July or August and see what the Colorado State Forest has to offer.

This forest actually abuts Rocky Mountain National Park, so that ought to give you an idea of the level of scenery here. North Park, the vast expanse of meadowland in Jackson County, is known as the moose capital of Colorado. Plan to see a few of those large critters and a few more animals if you explore the trails of Colorado State Forest.

After you drive that dizzying last mile to The Crags, take a deep breath and enter the campground. The setting is a high-country forest of subalpine fir and Engelmann spruce growing densely on steep slopes. Fear not, for the campsites have been leveled, though you may have to go up or down a bit to reach the camp from your car.

Don't drive too fast through the loop or you'll miss some of the campsites, which are set back in the woods. A few sites have pull-through areas for your vehicle, but don't expect to see any big rigs up here. That road discourages them, but any passenger car smaller than a moving truck can make the drive.

Enter a sunny area where you will see tree stumps left over from the days when this area was logged. Campsites here have a clear view of the severe lands above them. The loop reenters the woods and the more heavily wooded campsites begin. The last three campsites are very isolated and offer the most solitude.

RATINGS

Beauty: ✿ ✿ ✿
Privacy: ✿ ✿ ✿ ✿
Spaciousness: ✿ ✿ ✿
Quiet: ✿ ✿ ✿ ✿
Security: ✿ ✿ ✿
Cleanliness: ✿ ✿ ✿

Back at the beginning of the loop are vault toilets for each gender; the hand-pump well is to your left in the woods a bit. The water here is very cold.

Weekdays rarely find the camp filled. However, on later summer weekends, the campground will be alive with families and young couples, along with a few from the older generation who haven't converted to the dreaded RV. This hidden jewel of a park is not nearly as busy as other Front Range parks.

The Crags is close to some of the 71,000-acre Colorado State Forest's best hiking. Just up the road is the trail to Lake Agnes. It is less than a mile from the trailhead to the lake, which is banked against the Nokhu Crags. A path makes a loop around the lake. American Lakes are accessible by a 5-mile hike and offer views of the Medicine Bow Mountains. Make the one-way walk to Cameron Pass and have a shuttle car pick you up. Watchable wildlife includes mountain lions, elk, mule deer, coyote, and bear.

Ruby Jewel Lake is only a 1.5-mile trek. Kelly Lake and Clear Lake are other destination hikes in the park. If you fish these waters, remember that only artificial lures and flies are allowed. State regulations apply in park streams and in North Michigan Reservoir and Ranger Lakes.

Check out the Visitor Center with the unique barbed-wire moose outside and the stuffed moose inside. There are also informative displays on the park's wildlife that kids will really love.

In 1995, the Colorado Senate declared North Park "Moose Capital" of Colorado. Moose were introduced into North Park in the late 1970s and have been thriving here ever since. Try to observe moose in the early morning and late evening in the willow thickets along area creeks. You should also take the auto tour of the Arapaho National Wildlife Refuge in the heart of North Park. Get directions at the Visitor Center.

KEY INFORMATION

ADDRESS:	The Crags Campground Colorado State Forest 2746 Jackson County Road 41 Walden, CO 80480
OPERATED BY:	Colorado State Parks
INFORMATION:	(970) 723-8366; www.parks.state.co.us; state_forest@state.co.us
OPEN:	July–September
SITES:	26
EACH SITE HAS:	Picnic table, fire grate, tent pad
ASSIGNMENT:	By reservation or pick an available site on arrival
REGISTRATION:	(800) 678-CAMP (2267) or (303) 470-1144 in metro Denver; www.reserveamerica.com; at visitor center or park entrance
FACILITIES:	Vault toilets
PARKING:	At campsites only
FEE:	$5 Parks Pass plus $12 per night; an addition $8 fee added to each Internet or phone reservation
ELEVATION:	10,000 feet
RESTRICTIONS:	*Pets:* On leash only *Fires:* In fire grates only *Alcohol:* 3.2% beer only *Vehicles:* No trailers or motor homes allowed *Other:* 14-day stay limit in 45-day period

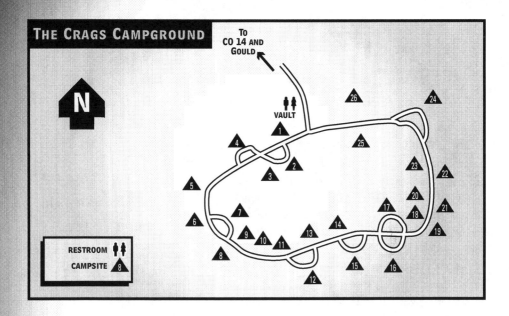

GETTING THERE

From Gould, drive north on CO 14 for 7 miles to FS 170. There will be a sign for Lake Agnes. Turn right on FS 170 and follow it for 0.5 mile to the first intersection. Turn right on FS 172 and climb steeply for 1 mile, turning left at the next intersection. Continue to The Crags Campground.

GPS COORDINATES

UTM Zone (WGS84)   13T
Easting   0423360
Northing   4482400
Latitude   N 40° 29' 19.3"
Longitude   W 105° 54' 14"

8
ELBERT CREEK CAMPGROUND

ACTIVE CAMPERS COME TO ELBERT CREEK, and it seems that they are not around enough to really take in the atmosphere of the campground. Elbert Creek has an agreeable location, high in the mountains along a resonant stream, where you really get a sense of being away from it all. But campers here seem to think they are near it all, at least those exercise-oriented pastimes that active campers like. Hiking is the main exercise; Mount Elbert and the Mount Massive Wilderness are just a walk away from the campground.

There are lakes and streams nearby for fishing. Mountain bikers like to pedal up to the Mount Champion Mill and the Colorado Trail, which is the backbone of the state's trail system. Somehow, campers find time to eat, sleep, and rest a little before going at it again the next day.

Elbert Creek is a small campground laid out underneath a lodgepole-pine forest in a flat along Halfmoon Creek. Enter the campground and the road splits into two drives running parallel to Halfmoon Creek that have vehicle turnarounds at their ends. This avails more streamside campsites. The forest is virtually devoid of ground cover, save for a few small saplings and rocks. However, the brush thickens alongside Halfmoon Creek, which flows loud and clear below the campground.

The right-hand drive has nine campsites. Many of these sites are spread far back in the woods. Four of the campsites are streamside and offer solitude. The left-hand drive has eight campsites that are very large, but three of them are a little close to the forest road that runs by the campground. Avoid the last three campsites unless you want to see who is driving by.

The pump well and vault toilets are conveniently in between the two drives. Elbert Creek receives heavy

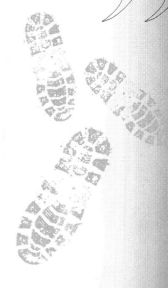

> *You can walk from your tent and hike up Mount Elbert, Colorado's highest peak at 14,433 feet.*

RATINGS

Beauty: ✪ ✪ ✪ ✪
Privacy: ✪ ✪ ✪
Spaciousness: ✪ ✪ ✪ ✪ ✪
Quiet: ✪ ✪ ✪
Security: ✪ ✪ ✪
Cleanliness: ✪ ✪ ✪

ADDRESS: Elbert Creek
Campground
Leadville Ranger
District
810 Front Street
Leadville, CO 80461

OPERATED BY: USDA Forest
Service, Pike and
San Isabel National
Forests, Cimarron
and Comanche
National Grasslands

INFORMATION: (719) 486-0749;
www.fs.fed.us/r2/
psicc/leadville

OPEN: June–Labor Day

SITES: 17

EACH SITE HAS: Picnic table, fire
grate

ASSIGNMENT: First come, first
served; no
reservation

REGISTRATION: Self-registration on
site

FACILITIES: Pump well, vault toilet, trash collection

PARKING: At campsites only

FEE: $12 per night

ELEVATION: 10,100 feet

RESTRICTIONS: *Pets:* On leash only
Fires: In fire grates
only
Alcohol: At campsites
only
Vehicles: 16 feet
Other: 14-day stay
limit

weekend use from hikers, so try to get there on Friday night or early Saturday if you are a weekend warrior. Otherwise, campsites are nearly always available.

Hikers love to bag peaks here in the Centennial State, and the highest point in Colorado, Mount Elbert, is very close. Elbert is the second highest point in the lower 48 states, behind Mount Whitney in California. It is a 3.5-mile climb to the crest from the nearby trail-head. There's nothing technical about this well-marked and maintained trail, though snow may present a prob-lem even in the early summer. You can also make a loop hike from here using the North Mount Elbert, South Mount Elbert, and Colorado Trails.

Just a short walk up the road is the Mount Mas-sive Wilderness. Much of this wilderness is above the timber line, so bring adequate clothing for inclement weather. Mount Massive is the second highest peak in Colorado, only 12 feet lower than Mount Elbert. You can stay at Elbert Creek and climb the two highest peaks in the state. Just beyond the Mount Elbert trail-head, take the Colorado Trail north into the wilderness up to the Mount Massive Trail and hike to the peak. You can also climb to the North Halfmoon Lakes using Trail 1485, which starts up FS 110 a couple of miles. Farther up this same road is the Champion Mine, with its aerial tramway still intact. You can bike or drive to the Champion Mine.

The Iron Mike Mine site is a hike or bike up South Halfmoon Creek. Nearby Emerald Lake features a picnic area and offers fishing, as do all the previously mentioned creeks. Speaking of fish, you ought to check out the Leadville National Fish Hatchery. Established in 1889, it is the second oldest federal fish hatchery in the country. Fish from here have been placed all over the Rockies, and today it still produces brook, cut-throat trout, and rainbow trout. There are trails on the hatchery grounds as well, with great views of the big mountains you came here to climb.

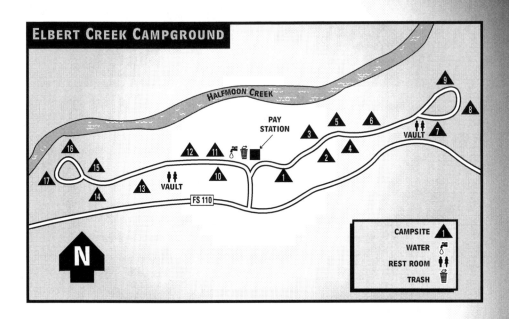

HALFMOON CREEK

PAY STATION

VAULT

VAULT

FS 110

N

CAMPSITE
WATER
REST ROOM
TRASH

GPS COORDINATES

UTM Zone (WGS84)	13S
Easting	0378500
Northing	4334880
Latitude	N 39° 9' 16.5"
Longitude	W 106° 24' 22"

GETTING THERE

From Leadville, head south on US 24 for 4 miles to CR 110 and the sign for the Leadville National Fish Hatchery. Turn right here and follow CR 110 for 0.7 mile to Halfmoon Creek Road. Turn left on Halfmoon Creek Road and follow it a short ways before the sharp right turn to stay on Halfmoon Creek Road. Continue on Halfmoon Creek Road as it turns to FS 110. Elbert Creek Campground will be 4 miles up on your right.

9
FLATIRON RESERVOIR CAMPGROUND

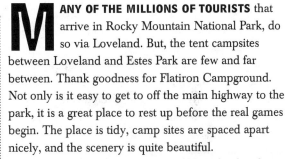

> *Great camping east of Rocky Mountain National Park and really the only option between Loveland, a main park gateway, and Estes Park.*

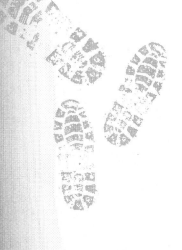

MANY OF THE MILLIONS OF TOURISTS that arrive in Rocky Mountain National Park, do so via Loveland. But, the tent campsites between Loveland and Estes Park are few and far between. Thank goodness for Flatiron Campground. Not only is it easy to get to off the main highway to the park, it is a great place to rest up before the real games begin. The place is tidy, camp sites are spaced apart nicely, and the scenery is quite beautiful.

The campground is just west of Loveland and is adjacent to Larimer County's Parks and Open Lands Carter Lake, Pinewood Lake, and Ramsay-Shockey Open Space. The landscape here is semi-arid with brush, small trees, red rock, and bluffs. Flatiron Reservoir itself includes 47 acres of water, plus 200 acres of public lands. This small lake is framed by Flatiron Mountain, a large, red bluff on the eastern side that towers over the water and the campground, which sits on the western waters edge.

If you are looking for a place to rest before or after you tackle Rocky Mountain National Park, this is the place. The other Larimer County open spaces in this area also provide camping access, but Flatiron Reservoir shines above them all. The campground is approximately 10 minutes from Loveland and about 40 minutes from Estes Park. The drive up the Thompson Canyon is a long crawl, especially during the summer months when campers are practically bumper to bumper up the winding road. If you can, time your visit in the early fall and not only will it cut your drive time, you may also be able to use Flatiron Campground as a base camp for exploring Rocky Mountain National Park.

Flatiron Campground lies along Flatiron Reservoir where boating and swimming are prohibited. Flatiron Mountain sits directly across the water and the arid landscape breaks up the rest of the campground.

RATINGS

Beauty: ✿ ✿ ✿
Privacy: ✿ ✿ ✿
Spaciousness: ✿ ✿ ✿
Quiet: ✿ ✿ ✿
Security: ✿ ✿ ✿ ✿
Cleanliness: ✿ ✿ ✿ ✿

Residential areas and the Flatiron Powerplant are adjacent to the campground but are not visible from most campsites. The first nine sites are adjacent to the group day-use area, but far enough from the water to offer some privacy. The host is here, and many of the smaller RVs tend to pick these spots. Continue up the main drive, and to the right is site F10 with large trees, plenty of shade and close to the water. Across the road is site F11 which looks like it gets the brunt of the traffic and wouldn't be my first pick.

Right before the main loop starts on a right spur, the main tent sites and cabins come up on the left and a good site, F12 sits to the right. I would consider all of the sites at Flatiron Campground to be good for tents, but these sites have walk-in access only. The two cabins look neat, are new, and each cabin also has an additional tent camp pad. The campsites F36 and F37 are similar, shaded, and close together, F35 is higher up on an overlook and does not offer much shade and appears to be very exposed.

Once the road spurs to the right, you enter the waterfront camping zone. The sites F13, F14, F16, F18, F20, F21, and F24 are all on the water and are very similar in that they have beautiful views, privacy, and plenty of space. Of the seven, F16 was my favorite. The sites across the road are nice, but a little more exposed; F19 is a handicapped-accessible site. Continuing on is another small spur that leads to two campsites (F26, F27) which offer good privacy. At the turn to these sites are two sites (F28, F25) that appear to be too close to the main County Road and were not that nice. Circle back along the loop and most of the sites here are higher up and more exposed. Site F33 is off to the side and hosts four large pines, F34 is in the middle section, but has some nice trees as well.

Flatiron Campground is open all year and many folks come here to trout fish, relax, or just picnic for the day. The Bison Visitor Center is close to the campground and has plenty of information on the area and tempts you with plenty of recreational activities. If you feel like getting cleaned up and spending money, an outlet shopping center and a new lifestyle mall sit on the far eastern edge of Loveland near I-25.

KEY INFORMATION

ADDRESS: Flatiron Reservoir Larimer County Parks and Open Lands Department 1800 South CR 31 Loveland, CO 80537

OPERATED BY: Larimer County

INFORMATION: (970) 679-4570; www .larimer.org/parks

OPEN: All year

SITES: 37, plus 2 camp cabins

EACH SITE HAS: Fire grate, picnic table

ASSIGNMENT: By reservation

REGISTRATION: (800) 397-7795 or www.larimer camping.com, or check in with camp host

FACILITIES: Vault toilets, water, wheelchair-accessible fishing pier, volleyball, horseshoe

PARKING: At sites or walk-in tent campers parking area

FEE: $12–$17 per night, plus $6–$7 entrance permit

ELEVATION: 5,470 feet

RESTRICTIONS: *Pets:* Leashed *Fires:* In designated grates only *Alcohol:* 3.2% beer permitted, glass prohibited *Vehicles:* 30 feet *Other:* Capacity varies by site; maximum 8 people in largest sites; no boating, 14-day stay limit; stay 100 feet away from dam; quiet hours 10 p.m.–6 a.m.

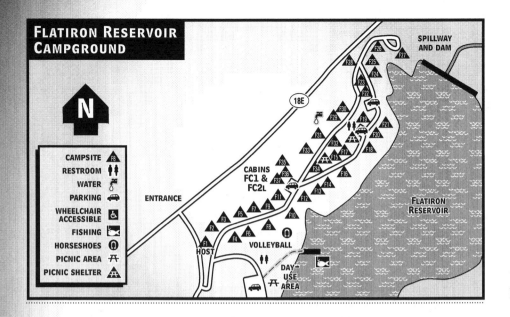

GETTING THERE

From Loveland, drive west on CO 34 to CR 29 (also known as Carter Lake Road). Turn right onto CR 18E, travel 2.6 miles, end at Flatiron Reservoir.

To get to Loveland, you probably drove north on I-25. If you want a change of pace, there are many areas along this Colorado Front Range corridor and into Wyoming that are accessible from Flatiron Campground. Go north to Fort Collins (30-minute drive) and enjoy the town or the outdoor recreation close to town. Horsetooth Reservoir, Lory State Park, and Poudre Canyon are honorable mentions. If you go south, you can sample the fun of Boulder (30-minute drive) or Denver (1-hour drive). Or, go even further north into Wyoming (1-hour drive) and open up a whole new world of western fun.

GPS COORDINATES

UTM Zone (WGS84)   13T
Easting   0480500
Northing   4468900
Latitude   N 39° 55' 10"
Longitude   W 105° 40' 40"

10
GENEVA PARK CAMPGROUND

GENEVA PARK CAMPGROUND was constructed by Forest Service volunteers in 1981. Not only did they produce a fine campground but they also chose their site well. The actual site is in a mildly rolling pine forest in the high country of the northern Pike National Forest. A mere 26 campsites are spread over a fair size of woodland. The location is ideal for exploring the Mount Evans Wilderness, which is less than a mile to the east.

At the head of the actual meadow of Geneva Park an unbroken stand of lodgepole pine grows. Their straight trunks, once used as tent poles for the lodges of western Indian tribes, form a beautiful sight when growing in dense stands as they do here at the campground. Most of the trees here don't have any branches on the lower part of their trunk, then they all seem to sprout branches lush with green needles, contrasting with their reddish-brown patterned bark. Their fallen needles lie on the ground, forming a dusky carpet among the scattered stones. I am sorry to report that some of these lodgepoles had to be cut down because of a dwarf mistletoe parasitic infestation, but the vast majority of trees remain to form an attractive landscape for your camping experience.

Cross Smelter Creek on a bridge, then come to the campground. Here, you will see the more open forest and some stumps of the trees that were cut down to keep the forest healthy. In spite of the cutting, the campsites here have adequate shade. These sites are closest to the pump well.

The actual loop begins after the first seven campsites. The road splits off to the right, just past the newly installed vault toilet. Campsites beneath the lodgepoles are either higher or lower than the road, depending on the variation of the terrain. As the loop swings around, there are three campsites that lie under the lodgepole

> *The Mount Evans Wilderness is just a hike away from Geneva Park.*

RATINGS

Beauty: ☆ ☆ ☆ ☆
Privacy: ☆ ☆ ☆
Spaciousness: ☆ ☆ ☆
Quiet: ☆ ☆ ☆ ☆
Security: ☆ ☆ ☆
Cleanliness: ☆ ☆ ☆

ADDRESS: Geneva Park
Campground
South Platte Ranger
District
19316 Goddard
Ranch Court
Morrison, CO 80465

OPERATED BY: USDA Forest
Service, Pike and
San Isabel National
Forests, Cimarron
and Comanche
National Grasslands

INFORMATION: (303) 275-5610;
www.fs.fed.us/r2/
psicc/spl

OPEN: May–October

SITES: 26

EACH SITE HAS: Picnic table, fire ring

ASSIGNMENT: First come, first
served; no
reservation

REGISTRATION: By phone (call (877)
444-6777), www
.reserveamerica
.com, or self-
registration on site

FACILITIES: Hand-pump well,
vault toilets

PARKING: At campsites only

FEE: $12 per night, an
additional $9 fee
added to each
phone or Internet
reservation

ELEVATION: 9,800 feet

RESTRICTIONS: *Pets:* On leash only
Fires: In fire rings
only
Alcohol: At campsites
only
Vehicles: 20 feet
Other: 14-day stay
limit

and border their own private meadow opposite the campground road. Beyond the meadow campsites, other campsites outside the loop climb up a hill.

This is the least used of the three campgrounds in the Geneva Creek valley. It normally doesn't fill on weekends or even most holidays. You should be able to get a campsite here on all but the busiest traditional holidays.

It's only a 15-minute walk to one of the trailheads to the Mount Evans Wilderness; it's a short drive to the other two entry points to the 74,000-acre preserve that was designated one year before Geneva Pass Campground came to be. Within the wilderness are two fourteeners and a rare type of arctic tundra, normally found only within the boundaries of the Arctic Circle. Small pools of water form a plant community unlike the normally dry, brittle Colorado alpine tundra. Mountain goats and bighorn sheep are at home here in this challenging environment.

There are three convenient points of entry to the wilderness for Geneva Park campers. Farther up CR 62 is Guanella Pass at 11,669 feet. It's the easiest way to get high. Just south of Geneva Park you will find the Abyss Trail commencement. This trail climbs strenuously along the glacier-carved valley of Scott Gomer Creek for seven miles to Abyss Lake. The lake lies perched in a cirque, an encircling wall of rock, with Mount Bierstadt on one side and Mount Evans on the other. Farther south on CR 62 is the Threemile Trail. It heads east into the wilderness toward Tahana Mountain and can be used in combination with the Rosalie and Abyss Trails to form a loop, if you don't mind a bit of road walking.

I enjoy camping in varied forest types. At Geneva Park you can have the lodgepole pine camping experience, then go have the Mount Evans Wilderness hiking experience.

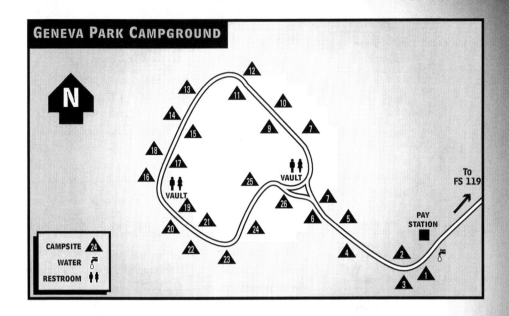

GENEVA PARK CAMPGROUND

N

12
13
11
10
14
9 7
15
18
17
16 VAULT VAULT
25
19 26
21 7
20 24 6 5
22 4
23 2
3

To
FS 119

PAY
STATION

CAMPSITE 24
WATER
RESTROOM

GETTING THERE

From US 285 in Grant, head
north on CR 62 toward
Guanella Pass for 6 miles,
then veer left on FS 119 and
follow it for 0.4 mile to
Geneva Park Campground,
which will be on your left.

GPS COORDINATES

UTM Zone (WGS84)   13S
Easting   0436490
Northing   4375280
Latitude   N 39° 31' 30.4"
Longitude   W 105° 44' 17"

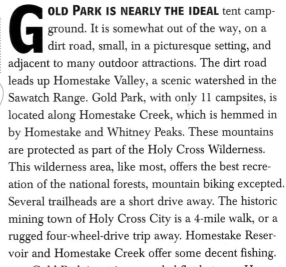

> *Mine yourself a good time at Gold Park.*

GOLD **PARK IS NEARLY THE IDEAL** tent campground. It is somewhat out of the way, on a dirt road, small, in a picturesque setting, and adjacent to many outdoor attractions. The dirt road leads up Homestake Valley, a scenic watershed in the Sawatch Range. Gold Park, with only 11 campsites, is located along Homestake Creek, which is hemmed in by Homestake and Whitney Peaks. These mountains are protected as part of the Holy Cross Wilderness. This wilderness area, like most, offers the best recreation of the national forests, mountain biking excepted. Several trailheads are a short drive away. The historic mining town of Holy Cross City is a 4-mile walk, or a rugged four-wheel-drive trip away. Homestake Reservoir and Homestake Creek offer some decent fishing.

Gold Park is set in a wooded flat between Homestake Creek and a low-lying hill covered in trees and boulders. Beyond the pay station the drive veers to the right, passing the campground host in the first campsite. Lodgepole pines and other smaller conifers shade the entire campsite. Large, spacious camping areas are spread along the loop as you proceed up the gravel drive, which then veers left as the rocky hill pinches in the flat toward the Homestake Creek.

The campsites come closer to the road as the vehicle turnaround approaches. Three of the best campsites are here, one snug against a shaded rock outcrop and the other two lying next to Homestake Creek. These last two campsites are the biggest and most coveted sites at Gold Park, which is a well-kept, clean campground.

Water spigots and a vault toilet serve this quaint camping area. Gold Park receives moderate use, filling up on the usual holidays. About the only RV you will see here is the campground host. It is unusual, but good, to have a host in a campground this small. The

RATINGS

Beauty: ✿ ✿ ✿ ✿ ✿
Privacy: ✿ ✿ ✿
Spaciousness: ✿ ✿ ✿ ✿ ✿
Quiet: ✿ ✿ ✿ ✿
Security: ✿ ✿ ✿ ✿
Cleanliness: ✿ ✿ ✿ ✿

mood here is serene, with the creek providing a naturally symphonic backdrop.

The upper part of this valley was once home to the mining town of Holy Cross City. The first mines were staked in 1880; Gold Park Mining Company was formed in 1881. The ore assays promised a boom. However, the outer layer of ore proved to be the richest, and the gold wasn't nearly as rich at deeper levels. By 1884, it was finally admitted that the mine was a bust. Another attempt was made in the same area in 1896; a deep tunnel was dug, but the profit just wasn't there. You can take FS 759 up to the site of this mine by foot, bike, or jeep. These days, your only strikes will be from fish on Homestake Creek or Homestake Reservoir, 3 miles up FS 703, your route to Gold Park. The lake is 480 acres in size and is brimming with trout.

Take time to explore the Holy Cross Wilderness, whose waters are coveted by Colorado Springs. However, development plans have been halted for the wilderness-that-almost-wasn't due to the city's tampering with the natural flows. Today, you can enjoy the wilderness's alpine lakes and icy streams. The Fall Creek Trail starts about 2 miles up the road to Holy Cross City. The trail heads up to Hunky Dory Lake and the stair-stepping Seven Sisters Lakes, where rock cliffs make for watery backdrops.

It's a 1,500-foot hike in 3 miles on the Missouri Lakes Trail. The trail starts up FS 704 and goes above the timber line. A shorter walk to a high-country lake is the Fancy Pass Trail, which also starts off of FS 704 above Gold Park. Pass some dams that you would be seeing all over the place if Colorado Springs had its way, then steeply make your way to Fancy Lake at 2 miles. Treasure Vault Lake is another mile beyond, though you have to go over Fancy Pass, and it is downhill to the lake.

Down from Gold Park is the Whitney Lake Trail, which offers views on its 2.3-mile journey to Whitney Lake. From here you can scale 13,271-foot Mount Whitney, rising on the north shore of the lake, if you follow the west ridge to the top. No matter where you go in the Holy Cross Wilderness, appreciate it, because it almost never came into existence.

KEY INFORMATION

ADDRESS:	Gold Park Campground Holy Cross Ranger District 24747 US 24 Minturn, CO 81645
OPERATED BY:	USDA Forest Service, White River National Forest
INFORMATION:	(970) 827-5715; www.wildernet.com
OPEN:	May–September
SITES:	11
EACH SITE HAS:	Picnic table, fire grate
ASSIGNMENT:	First come, first served; no reservation
REGISTRATION:	Self-registration on site
FACILITIES:	Water spigot, vault toilets, trash collection
PARKING:	At campsites only
FEE:	$12 per night
ELEVATION:	9,300 feet
RESTRICTIONS:	*Pets:* On leash only *Fires:* In fire grates only *Alcohol:* At campsites only *Vehicles:* 40 feet *Other:* 10-day stay limit

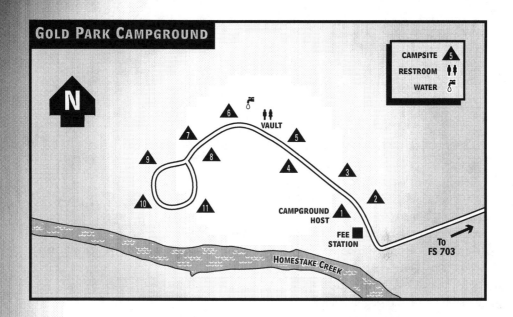

GETTING THERE

From I-70 near Minturn, head south on US 24 for 11.5 miles to FS 703 (Homestake Road). Turn right on FS 703 and follow it for 7 miles to Gold Park Campground, which will be on your left.

GPS COORDINATES

UTM Zone (WGS84)   13S
Easting   0376420
Northing   4362660
Latitude   N 39° 24' 16.0"
Longitude   W 106° 26' 7.3"

12
GOLDEN GATE CANYON STATE PARK CAMPGROUND

GOLDEN **GATE IS A PRESERVED SLICE** of the Rocky Mountains just a few minutes away from Denver. Rock spires stand out among rich forests and green meadows. Vistas offer outstanding views of the Continental Divide to the west. Well-marked and well-maintained trails meander down watery glens to open meadows, where settlements once stood. This refuge is rich in wildlife, from birds to bears. With 55 walk-in tent sites, your camping experience promises to be a good one.

There are two primary campgrounds at Golden Gate Canyon. Reverends Ridge is the big one; it offers spaces for every type of camper. There are ten camp loops of every shape and description, including small circles with parking areas radiating like spokes. There are two loops with pull-through sites for RVs. The old group campground has been converted to six mini-loops that can only be described as different.

But tent campers need only concern themselves with loops F, G, and J in Reverends Ridge; these offer walk-in tent sites. Loops F and G are next to each other. It is a short walk from the parking area to your tent site beneath the lodgepole pines or an aspen grove or two. Loop J is at the very end of the main camping drive, cutting down on drive-by traffic. Some of the campsites are close to the parking area; others are set back in the woods. A stay at Reverends Ridge offers tent campers a compromise: you can stay at the tent sites and still access the water spigots and the hot showers and flush toilets located in the camper services building.

Aspen Meadow, on the other hand, is more rustic and is the preferred area for tent campers. It has hand-pump wells and vault toilets. But it is also more scenic and isolated from the rest of the campground. Aspen Meadow itself is broken up into three distinctive walk-in tent camping areas.

> *This tent-camping getaway is only 30 miles from the Denver metropolitan area.*

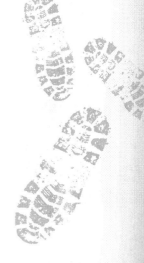

RATINGS

Beauty: ✪ ✪ ✪
Privacy: ✪ ✪ ✪
Spaciousness: ✪ ✪ ✪
Quiet: ✪ ✪ ✪
Security: ✪ ✪ ✪ ✪ ✪
Cleanliness: ✪ ✪ ✪ ✪

ADDRESS: Golden Gate Canyon State Park 92 Crawford Gulch Road Golden, CO 80403

OPERATED BY: Colorado State Parks

INFORMATION: (303) 582-3707 or (303) 642-3856 in the summer; www.parks .state.co.us

OPEN: Aspen Meadow Loop, all year; Reverends Ridge Loop, May–October

SITES: 55 walk-in tent sites, 86 other

EACH SITE HAS: Picnic table, fire grate, tent pad

ASSIGNMENT: By reservation or on site

REGISTRATION: (800) 678-CAMP (2267) or (303) 470-1144 in metro Denver, www.reserve america.com

FACILITIES: Hot showers, flush and vault toilets, laundry, phone, vending; 28 sites have electricity

PARKING: At campsites or walk-in tent campers parking area

FEE: $5 Parks Pass plus $12 per night walk-in tent sites at Aspen Meadows or Reverends Ridge; $16 for electrical hookups; $8 added to each reservation

ELEVATION: 9,100 feet

RESTRICTIONS: *Pets:* On leash only
Fires: In fire grates only
Alcohol: 3.2% beer only
Vehicles: 40 feet
Other: 14-day stay limit in 45-day period

The Meadow Loop has 14 campsites in a conifer and aspen wood, next to a large meadow. The campsites on one side of the dirt road are situated amid large boulders that add to the character of the area. The Twin Creek and Conifer Loops are off the ridge in a small valley. The woods are denser here, and a small stream adds to the setting. These are the most popular tent-only sites and are the first to be claimed. Some of the campsites are nearly 100 yards away from the parking area.

The Rimrock Loop has several wooded campsites up on a ridge punctuated with boulder landscaping; these sites offer a view of the lands in the distance. These campsites also have the pump well nearest to them. Vault toilets are set in each loop at Aspen Meadow.

No matter where you camp, reservations are highly recommended and practically mandatory for summer weekends. Go ahead and make the call to ensure yourself a preferred campsite. Weekdays are not such a problem in this safe, family-oriented campground and natural area.

While you are in the campground, check the notices about ranger programs that are held nightly on weekends. You can learn about the human and natural history of the park in these talks led by park naturalists. There are kids' programs on weekend days that cater specifically to young campers who want to have a good time and learn something about nature without feeling like they are in school.

Other campers will want to strike out on their own on some of the 35 miles of park trails. Everyone should walk the Raccoon Trail. It begins at Panorama Point, where you have a fantastic view of the Continental Divide, and it has interpretive signs to teach hikers a thing or two. The most popular loop hike is the Mountain Lion Trail, which winds for 7 miles into Forgotten Valley, back up a canyon, and up by Windy Peak. Take the side trail to the top of Windy Peak.

The walk into Frazer Meadow is one of the more picturesque park settings. There are three ways to get to the meadow, including the Mule Deer Trail, which connects to Aspen Meadows Campground. There are

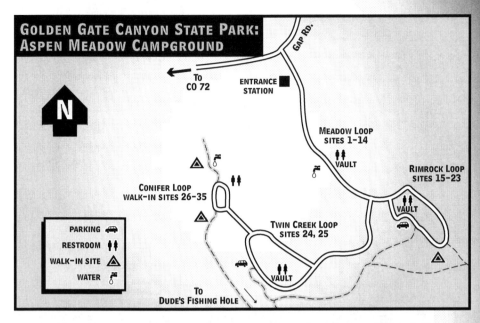

GOLDEN GATE CANYON STATE PARK:
ASPEN MEADOW CAMPGROUND

GAP RD.

To
CO 72

ENTRANCE
STATION

N

MEADOW LOOP
SITES 1-14

VAULT

RIMROCK LOOP
SITES 15-23

CONIFER LOOP
WALK-IN SITES 26-35

VAULT

TWIN CREEK LOOP
SITES 24, 25

PARKING
RESTROOM
WALK-IN SITE
WATER

VAULT

To
DUDE'S FISHING HOLE

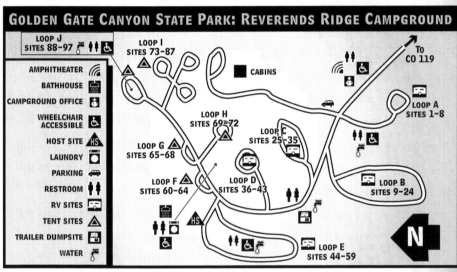

GOLDEN GATE CANYON STATE PARK: REVERENDS RIDGE CAMPGROUND

LOOP J
SITES 88-97

LOOP I
SITES 73-87

To
CO 119

AMPHITHEATER
BATHHOUSE
CAMPGROUND OFFICE
WHEELCHAIR
ACCESSIBLE
HOST SITE
LAUNDRY
PARKING
RESTROOM
RV SITES
TENT SITES
TRAILER DUMPSITE
WATER

CABINS

LOOP A
SITES 1-8

LOOP H
SITES 69-72

LOOP C
SITES 25-35

LOOP G
SITES 65-68

LOOP F
SITES 60-64

LOOP D
SITES 36-43

LOOP B
SITES 9-24

N

LOOP E
SITES 44-59

five ponds in the park and a few small streams that offer trout fishing. Dude's Fishing Hole is very near Aspen Meadows. Denverites and visitors should take advantage of this quick getaway to the real, natural Colorado.

GPS COORDINATES

UTM Zone (WGS84)	13S
Easting	0463240
Northing	4409570
Latitude	N 39° 50' 7.4"
Longitude	W 105° 25' 6.0"

GETTING THERE

From Golden, take CO 93 north for 1 mile to Golden Gate Canyon Road. Turn left and follow Golden Gate Canyon Road for 15 miles to the park.

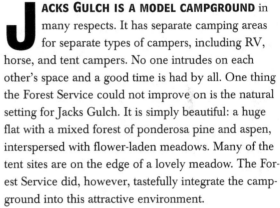

> *Jacks Gulch is the forest campground of the future. It has a little bit of something for everyone, including ten attractive walk-in tent sites.*

JACKS **G**ULCH **IS A MODEL CAMPGROUND** in many respects. It has separate camping areas for separate types of campers, including RV, horse, and tent campers. No one intrudes on each other's space and a good time is had by all. One thing the Forest Service could not improve on is the natural setting for Jacks Gulch. It is simply beautiful: a huge flat with a mixed forest of ponderosa pine and aspen, interspersed with flower-laden meadows. Many of the tent sites are on the edge of a lovely meadow. The Forest Service did, however, tastefully integrate the campground into this attractive environment.

Enter Jacks Gulch Campground on the main road. Off to your right is the Equestrian Camp. There are five sites with the same amenities as the regular campsites, except they each have a minicorral for the horses. The sites are large and spread farther apart than the average campsites. The two group campgrounds are also over this way.

Veer left, then stay straight and come to the Yarrow Loop. Nice campsites with the newest grills, grates, tent pads, and picnic tables add to the naturally appealing setting. All manner of campers can enjoy this loop, where most of the campsites are shaded by large ponderosa pines.

The other loop is the Columbine Loop; it weaves around like a snake. The campsites have electrical hookups in addition to the standard amenities. This is the home of the big rigs. Splintering off this loop, however, is the walk-in tent camper's area. There is a water spigot and vault toilet in the parking area for tent campers to use. Follow a little gravel path away from the parking area into an aspen wood mixed with some conifers. The campsites themselves splinter off from the main gravel path on a gravel path of their own. Each campsite is far from its neighbor. It's almost like

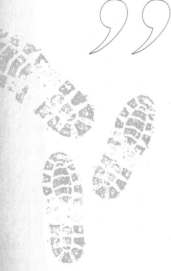

RATINGS

Beauty: ✩ ✩ ✩ ✩ ✩
Privacy: ✩ ✩ ✩ ✩
Spaciousness: ✩ ✩ ✩ ✩
Quiet: ✩ ✩ ✩ ✩
Security: ✩ ✩ ✩ ✩
Cleanliness: ✩ ✩ ✩ ✩

each site is its own miniature campground. I highly recommend this tent-camping experience.

The first five sites have a path of their own, and the second five campsites have their own path as well. Each of these paths connects to the gravel Campground Loop Trail, which makes for a good morning leg-stretcher.

Up Flowers Road beyond the campground is the Flowers Trail. You may have to walk part of the four-wheel-drive road to get to it. After intersecting Beaver Park, enter the Comanche Peaks Wilderness. Elk roam this wilderness, which is also known for its fishing. Leave Beaver Park and climb up to Browns Lake. This path was an old wagon trail in the 1800s.

Little Beaver Creek Trail and Fish Creek Trail enter the wilderness just a little south of the campground on CR 44H. Both make moderate ascents up their respective watersheds and offer trout fishing for hikers and horseback riders. Other trails enter the wilderness from forest roads south of Jacks Gulch. Consult your Arapaho and Roosevelt National Forest map, which you should buy before coming to Jacks Gulch. Not too far south is the northern border of Rocky Mountain National Park, which can be accessed by foot from Pingree Park up the Mummy Pass Trail.

You can also make Jacks Gulch a base camp for recreating in the Poudre Canyon. Rafters, kayakers, and anglers are seen in and around the river, testing the waters. This campground is much more desirable than those in the canyon, yet it is only 6 miles from the canyon and river. You can leave the crowded canyon with its roadside campgrounds and return to Jacks Gulch, where the scene is much quieter and the camping is some of the best in the state.

ADDRESS: Jacks Gulch Campground Canyon Lakes Ranger District 2150 Centre Avenue, Building E Fort Collins, CO 80526

OPERATED BY: USDA Forest Service, Arapaho and Roosevelt National Forests, Pawnee National Grassland

INFORMATION: (970) 295-6700; www.fs.fed.us/r2/arnf

OPEN: May 19– November 13

SITES: 10 walk-in tent only, 5 equestrian, 55 other

EACH SITE HAS: Picnic table, fire grate, stand-up grill, tent pad

ASSIGNMENT: First come, first served; no reservation; 2 equestrian sites reservable at www.reserveusa.com

REGISTRATION: Register with host

FACILITIES: Water spigots, vault toilets, some sites have electricity

PARKING: At campsites and walk-in tent parking area

FEE: $15; $5 for electricity; $25 equestrian sites plus $9 reservation fee

ELEVATION: 8,100 feet

RESTRICTIONS: *Pets:* On leash only; see Web for specific horse restrictions *Fires:* In fire grates *Alcohol:* At sites *Vehicles:* 50 feet *Other:* 14-day limit

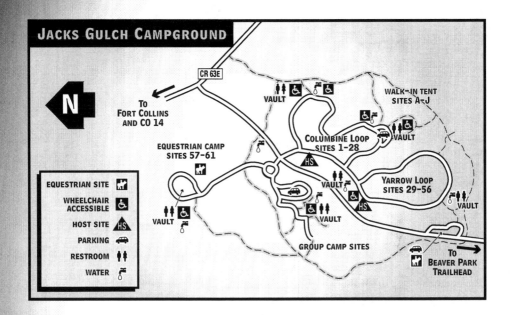

GETTING THERE

From Fort Collins, drive 10 miles north on US 287 to CO 14. Turn left on CO 14 (Poudre Canyon Highway) and follow it for 24 miles to CR 63E (Pingree Park Road). You will see a sign for Pingree Park. Turn left on CR 63E and follow it for 6 miles to Jacks Gulch Campground, which will be on your right.

GPS COORDINATES

UTM Zone (WGS84)   13T
Easting   0455270
Northing   4497413
Latitude   N 40° 37' 35.0"
Longitude   W 105° 31' 43.0"

14
LONGS PEAK CAMPGROUND

LONGS PEAK CAMPGROUND offers the best and worst of the American national park system. This tents-only camping area is located in a scenic setting adjacent to some of the most beautiful mountain land in the Rockies. There are many sights to see and things to do, but the very things that attract you to this park also attract many other visitors.

Longs Peak is an extremely popular hike here. Cars will line the road leading to the trailhead and campground. It takes a combination of timing and luck to get a campsite during the peak season, which is from late June through mid-September. When you do get a campsite, you will realize that in spite of all the cars nearby, the hustle and bustle won't overwhelm you in this 26-site campground. The trailhead parking area, however, will have all the hustle and bustle.

Pass the line of parked cars along Longs Peak Road and come to a split in the road. Turn right and enter the campground. To your left is the always-full-during-the-summer trailhead parking. The teardrop-shaped, gravel campground loop makes its way beneath a lodgepole woodland pocked with boulders and smaller trees. The campsites are mostly on the outside of the loop and have somewhat obstructed views of the Twin Sisters peaks across the Tahosa Valley in the Roosevelt National Forest.

More campsites are stretched along the peak side of the loop. As popular as they are, they are well maintained. A hill rises against the campground. This is the campground's rockier side; campsites are more spread out over here. Overall, the sites are average in size, with ample room for the average tent. But always being full does make the place seem a bit confined. Colorful tents and colorful people give Longs Peak some extra pizzazz.

> *This tent-only campground can be your base camp for exploring the east side of Rocky Mountain National Park.*

RATINGS

Beauty: ☆ ☆ ☆
Privacy: ☆ ☆
Spaciousness: ☆ ☆ ☆
Quiet: ☆ ☆
Security: ☆ ☆ ☆ ☆
Cleanliness: ☆ ☆ ☆ ☆

KEY INFORMATION

ADDRESS: Longs Peak
Campground
Rocky Mountain
National Park
Estes Park, CO 80517

OPERATED BY: National Park
Service; Rocky
Mountain National
Park

INFORMATION: (970) 586-1206;
www.nps.gov/romo

OPEN: All year

SITES: 26

EACH SITE HAS: Picnic table, fire
grate, tent pad

ASSIGNMENT: First come, first
served; no
reservation

REGISTRATION: Self-registration on
site

FACILITIES: Water spigot, flush
toilets (no water
October–May)

PARKING: At campsites only

FEE: $20 per night
(Memorial Day–
mid-September) or
$14 in the off season
when the water is
shut off; plus a
separate park
entrance fee applies

ELEVATION: 9,400 feet

RESTRICTION: *Pets:* On leash only
Fires: In fire grates
only
Alcohol: At campsites
only
Vehicles: No RVs
Other: 7 nights per
campsite; 14-night
limit in winter

Water spigots are situated around the campground, but there is only one toilet for each gender located in the center of the campground. You might have to wait in line for that too. Realistically, you will feel lucky and appreciative when you do get a campsite; you'll still have a pleasurable tent camping experience here. Try to get here on the shoulder seasons—June or late September—and you can get a campsite much easier. Bring your own water and a warm sleeping bag if you come in winter.

I recommend auto-touring the park your first day, maybe doing some shorter hikes, then tackling Longs Peak first thing the next morning, when you have all day to make the climb. Driving Trail Ridge Road is a must. It is a rite of passage at Rocky Mountain National Park. The views are as exhilarating as the air is cold up there. Then check out the exhibits and self-guiding nature trail at Moraine Park Museum. Back at Longs Peak, take a warm-up hike on the Storm Pass Trail. It leads up to the Eugenia Mine Site and onto Storm Pass after 2.5 miles.

Then go to bed early. Your route to the top of Longs Peak will be the Keyhole Route, which is generally free of snow from mid-July until mid-September. The final part of the route is 1.6 miles beyond the end of the maintained trail; most of the scramble is marked on the rock below you.

The park service recommends that you try to leave the trailhead between 3 a.m. and 6 a.m. to make the 7.5 miles to the summit of Longs Peak by noon. Bad weather can arise at any time, but it is more likely in the afternoon during the summer. Bring plenty of warm clothes and plenty of lung power. The round trip lasts from 12 to 15 hours. Make sure and keep your campsite a second night because you will be too exhausted to do anything except make supper and hit the sack.

Just a few miles south of Longs Peak is the Wild Basin area, a quieter section of the park's east side. Many old-time Rocky Mountain enthusiasts consider this to be the best area of the park. There are many watery features in the basin that make great day hikes. It is only 0.3 miles from the Ranger Station in Wild Basin to Copeland Falls. Calypso Cascades is 1.8 miles up

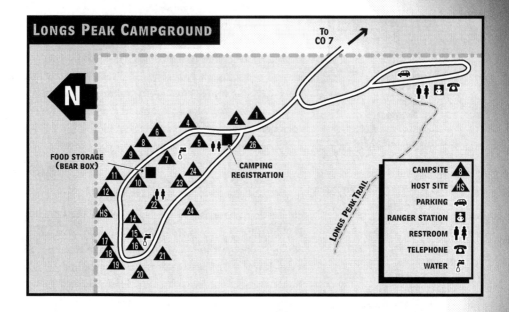

LONGS PEAK CAMPGROUND

To CO 7

N

FOOD STORAGE
(BEAR BOX)

CAMPING
REGISTRATION

LONGS PEAK TRAIL

CAMPSITE	8
HOST SITE	HS
PARKING	🚗
RANGER STATION	🏠
RESTROOM	🚻
TELEPHONE	☎
WATER	🚰

where Saint Vrain Creek splits. Ouzel Falls is 2.7 miles up the trail from the Ranger Station. Continue a little farther to see the peaks above and the plains below. There are several alpine lakes to access in Wild Basin.

GETTING THERE

From Estes Park, head south on CO 7 for 8 miles to Longs Peak Road. Turn right on Longs Peak Road and follow it for 3 miles to Longs Peak Campground, which will be on your right.

GPS COORDINATES

UTM Zone (WGS84)	13T
Easting	0452520
Northing	4458400
Latitude	N 40° 16' 29.5"
Longitude	W 105° 33' 9.0"

15
LOST PARK
CAMPGROUND

> *Lost Park is your camping ticket to the Lost Creek Wilderness.*

LOST **P**ARK **C**AMPGROUND sits atop a knoll in the large valley at the confluence of Indian Creek, North Fork Lost Creek, and South Fork Lost Creek. The Kenosha and Tarryall Mountains serve as your campground cathedrals. It is in this enhanced setting that you can set up your tent, then fish, hike, and explore the Lost Creek Wilderness until the call of civilization is too loud to ignore.

You won't want to leave this small, hilltop campground cloaked in lodgepole pines and complemented by other conifers. With only 12 campsites and nearly 20 miles of dirt road, civilization doesn't exactly come knocking on your tent flap. Two drives with vehicle turnarounds at their ends divide the campsites, which are spread very far apart.

The first drive circles the top of the knoll. Most of the campsites are on the more heavily wooded left side, while the few on the right look over Lost Creek below and Bison Peak above. A campsite lies in the rocky center of the auto turnaround. Other boulders serve as landscaping car barriers.

The lower drive turns left and drops toward the North Fork of Lost Creek. Two campsites lie on a slope to your left. Stay here if you don't mind sleeping a little tilted. Pass the northbound section of the Brookside-McCurdy Trail. Follow the drive as it swings right along the creek, passing the well pump in a meadow and a lonesome campsite on your right that offers the maximum in privacy. The drive continues past other campsites that sit on a small hill looking downstream on Lost Creek. These sites also have other conifers in addition to the lodgepole. Then you come to the vehicle turnaround with one more large campsite on your right.

There is one set of vault toilets for each gender at each loop. But bigger amenities, such as three fishable streams and three trailheads at the campground, will

RATINGS

Beauty: ✩ ✩ ✩ ✩
Privacy: ✩ ✩ ✩ ✩
Spaciousness: ✩ ✩ ✩ ✩
Quiet: ✩ ✩ ✩ ✩
Security: ✩ ✩ ✩
Cleanliness: ✩ ✩ ✩

make you appreciate Lost Park more than anything else. The Lost Creek Wilderness, which is most of the land you see around you, is almost 120,000 acres of meadows, woods, and unusual granite formations, where one of Colorado's largest herds of bighorn sheep live. There are nearly 100 miles of trails to enjoy, and you probably can get most of the hiking you desire without restarting your vehicle until it is time to head home. After all, a wilderness is defined as an untrammeled place where man is just a visitor. And visit you must.

The Wigwam Trail heads east along Lost Creek proper. Soon you'll come to the very large East Lost Park. This is a huge meadow that goes on and on. Veer right on an unmaintained fishing trail if you want to keep going down Lost Creek. The Wigwam Trail follows a feeder stream up and over a divide to the Wigwam Creek drainage.

The north end of the Brookside-McCurdy Trail skirts the wilderness; mountain bikers can pedal this section. It then intersects the Colorado Trail, where you can veer right into the wilderness high country or veer left and keep on biking to the top, over to the Craig Creek drainage. If you go south on the Brookside-McCurdy Trail from the campground, you will head up Indian Creek toward Bison Pass. There are fishable waters with small, but spunky trout ready to tear at your lure on all the creeks.

Mountain bikers can't enter the wilderness, but they have their own trails to use just back down FS 56. Walleye Gulch Road and Topaz Road, FS 854 and FS 446, respectively, can be used with other connecting Forest Service roads to make loops. I recommend that hikers, bikers, and anglers all get the Trails Illustrated map titled "Tarryall Mountains, Kenosha Pass," for the general area (**maps.nationalgeographic.com/trails**). Get all your supplies before you get anywhere near the area; Lost Park is far from the main roads. The nearby towns are small and don't have much in the way of supplies except for the convenience store variety. One more thing, bring your binoculars to help you spot bighorn sheep.

KEY INFORMATION

ADDRESS: Lost Park Campground South Park Ranger District P.O. Box 219 320 Highway 285 Fairplay, CO 80440

OPERATED BY: USDA Forest Service, Pike and San Isabel National Forests, Cimarron and Comanche National Grasslands

INFORMATION: (719) 836-2031; www.fs.fed.us/r2/psicc/sopa

OPEN: May–September

SITES: 12

EACH SITE HAS: Picnic table, fire grate

ASSIGNMENT: First come, first served; no reservation

REGISTRATION: Self-registration on site

FACILITIES: Hand-pump well, vault toilets

PARKING: At campsites only

FEE: $7 per night

ELEVATION: 10,000 feet

RESTRICTIONS: *Pets:* On leash only *Fires:* In fire grates only *Alcohol:* At campsites only *Vehicles:* 22 feet *Other:* 14-day stay limit

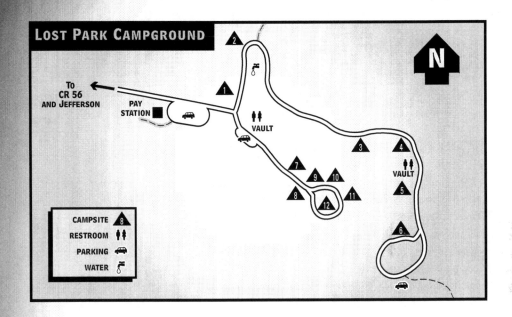

GETTING THERE

From Jefferson, drive north
1 mile to CR 56 (Lost
Park Road), turn right and
drive east for 19 miles to
the dead end at Lost Park
Campground.

GPS COORDINATES

UTM Zone (WGS84)   13S
Easting   0456350
Northing   4348440
Latitude   N 39° 17' 4.0"
Longitude   W 105° 30 22.0"

16
LOWER NARROWS CAMPGROUND

THE POUDRE (pronounced: pooh-der) River is full of plenty of river lore and conjures up images of French trappers hooting down fierce rapids in the canyon. Its official name is Cache la Poudre River and legend has it that the river was named when a party of westward furtrappers were forced to lighten their load near the banks after being caught in a heavy snowfall. The order was given to "cache la poudre" or "hide the powder" so that it could be retrieved the following spring. The Poudre River, with it's designation as a Wild and Scenic River, is quite wild. In heavy run-off years, we've rafted sections of the river that spilled us in and claimed this author, hooting and hollering, bobbing along, until pulled back inside our boat. Luckily I emerged unscathed, but the river earns quick respect from those who recreate here. One area that is sacred is a section called the Narrows: a narrow cleft where the river has cut through the rock walls. Even driving through this area is dicey, with hairpin turns, blind spots, and looming canyon walls. If I want a good scare, we park and look at the river during the spring, when the water is crashing down, full of the cold, spring run off. The Class VI rapids tear into the canyon walls and pummel anything in their path. A few crazies and experienced kayakers have been known to run these rapids and live to tell. (River rapids are usually rated on a raftable scale starting at I, considered easy and ending at V, considered not so easy. So you get the idea on what a VI means.)

The Narrows Campgrounds, both Upper and Lower are located just above said rapids. From the Lower Narrows campground, you can walk a half-mile to witness the gnarly area previously described.

Poudre Canyon recreationists are usually limited to RV clogged camping areas with one exception. The Lower Narrows is the tent only portion of the Narrows

> *The Lower Narrows, right on a wild river, is the best tent camping in the canyon.*

RATINGS

Beauty: ☆ ☆ ☆
Privacy: ☆ ☆ ☆
Spaciousness: ☆ ☆ ☆
Quiet: ☆ ☆ ☆
Security: ☆ ☆ ☆ ☆
Cleanliness: ☆ ☆ ☆ ☆ ☆

ADDRESS: Lower Narrows
Canyon Lakes
Ranger District
2150 Centre Avenue,
Building E
Fort Collins, CO
80526

OPERATED BY: USDA Forest
Service, Arapaho
and Roosevelt
National Forests,
Pawnee National
Grassland

INFORMATION: (970) 295-6700;
www.fs.fed.us/r2/arnf

OPEN: May–October

SITES: 8

EACH SITE HAS: Fire grate, picnic
table, tent pad

ASSIGNMENT: By reservation

REGISTRATION: By phone (877) 444-
6777, online at www
.reserveusa.com, or
self-registration on
site

FACILITIES: Vault toilets, drinking water (usually
turned off at the end
of September)

PARKING: Lot for exactly 8 cars

FEE: $14 (half price when
water is not avail-
able), an additional
$9 fee added to each
Internet or phone
reservation

ELEVATION: 6,400 feet

RESTRICTIONS: *Pets:* On leash
Fires: In grates
Alcohol: Allowed
Vehicles: Passenger
vehicles only
Other: 8 people per
site

Campground, complete with a separate entrance and is by far the best tent camping in the canyon. There is plenty of hiking, especially in the nearby Comanche Peak Wilderness. Anglers, off-road enthusiasts, and Sunday drivers all clog the roadway, especially during the summer weekends, but they all seem to be having a great time. The Poudre River is the main draw to the Narrows Campground and the Lower Narrows camp-sites are as close as you can get to sleeping on shore, especially preferred sites 12 and 13. Site 14 is a good second choice and site 11 isn't bad either but it is a lit-tle higher from the river. Light sleepers take note, the river rages through here in May and June with accom-panying noise.

Lower Narrows Campground is configured as a loop. At the entrance, take a right turn to start a counter clockwise loop. Numbering starts at site 8 since Lower Narrows and Upper Narrows are man-aged jointly by the ranger district at the Narrows Campground. Park at the parking lot right next to site 8. There is an obvious disadvantage to being near the parking lot. Site 8, along with sites 9 and 10 are closer to the road. Sites 11 through 15 are scattered about from here. As mentioned before, sites 12 and 13 are most popular, with 14 not far behind and sites 11 and 15 earning honorable mentions.

Even in other months this is not a sleepy stretch of river, but a rather steep and rocky section, as is most of Poudre Canyon. The river may be boated by experi-enced rafters and kayakers above this area and again resuming at Stevens Gulch, 2.5 miles downstream. Between the campground and Stevens Gulch are the several Class VI drops hidden from the road. Lower Narrows campground is a good alternative to the high use, RV-type campgrounds in the area. There are very little services for miles in either direction except for a few seasonal stores. If you are interested in rafting or kayaking, the Poudre River is open to both private and commercial boaters. We have our own gear, but would recommend setting up an outfitted trip in Fort Collins before heading out.

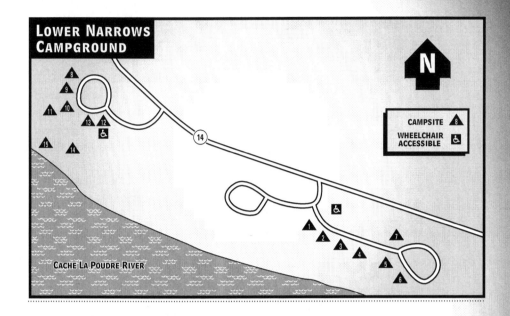

LOWER NARROWS CAMPGROUND

CACHE LA POUDRE RIVER

N

CAMPSITE 8
WHEELCHAIR ACCESSIBLE ♿

GETTING THERE

Drive 7 miles north of Fort Collins on US 287. Turn left on CO 14, drive approximately 16 miles west on CO 14, also known as Poudre Canyon Highway. If coming from upper Poudre Canyon/Cameron Pass, look for the entrance just after Narrows Campground.

GPS COORDINATES

UTM Zone (WGS84) 13T
Easting 0463318
Northing 4503812
Latitude N 40° 41' 21.2"
Longitude W 105° 25' 57"

17
PEACEFUL VALLEY AND CAMP DICK CAMPGROUNDS

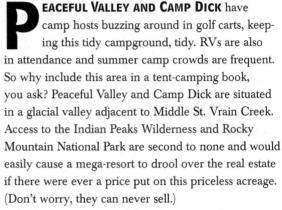

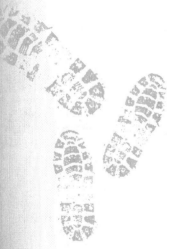

> *The access to Indian Peaks Wilderness and Rocky Mountain National Park is second to none.*

PEACEFUL VALLEY AND CAMP DICK have camp hosts buzzing around in golf carts, keeping this tidy campground, tidy. RVs are also in attendance and summer camp crowds are frequent. So why include this area in a tent-camping book, you ask? Peaceful Valley and Camp Dick are situated in a glacial valley adjacent to Middle St. Vrain Creek. Access to the Indian Peaks Wilderness and Rocky Mountain National Park are second to none and would easily cause a mega-resort to drool over the real estate if there were ever a price put on this priceless acreage. (Don't worry, they can never sell.)

The arrangement of the 58 campsites here is carefully thought out with particular attention paid to placement of the campsites tucked into the wooded landscape. All campers live in harmony here, especially those confined to the smaller sites. RV campers may also convert to smaller accommodations after visiting when they see what amazing spots are allowed for tent campers here.

Technically two campgrounds, Peaceful Valley and Camp Dick are connected by a short road and appear to be one and the same. The access to scenery and recreation opportunities in Indian Peaks Wilderness and Rocky Mountain National Park is the reason to be here. Hiking can even be directly accessed from the St. Vrain trailhead at the west end of the campsite. Backpackers, horseback riders, mountain bikers, four-wheel-drive users, and anglers all enjoy the advantages of the surroundings. Since Indian Peaks is a wilderness area, those wanting to camp there or recreate in the wilderness boundary should contact the Boulder Ranger District regarding specific regulations that apply. The same goes for Rocky Mountain National Park, so contact the National Park Service for rules particular to that area. It's important to note that without entering

RATINGS

Beauty: ✿ ✿ ✿ ✿
Privacy: ✿ ✿ ✿
Spaciousness: ✿ ✿ ✿ ✿
Quiet: ✿ ✿ ✿
Security: ✿ ✿ ✿ ✿
Cleanliness: ✿ ✿ ✿ ✿

the wilderness or national park, there is plenty to do. The campground itself is still in the national forests.

Peaceful Valley and Camp Dick have been remodeled recently and the biggest improvement is the paved road that cuts down on dust creeping into the campsites. Some sites at Peaceful Valley and Camp Dick are not recommended during peak season because of privacy and the fact that they are essentially set up for RVs. But the cream of the crop, mentioned here, are nice, especially if you can get here during the weekdays. Of the 58 campsites, we have made a list of the top ten. By far the best for privacy and space is Camp Dick site 35 at the end of a loop. Camp Dick sites 10, 12, 15, 16, 18, 19, 40, and 41 are also recommended for space and privacy. Peaceful Valley site 1 is the final pick because a slight embankment provides extra privacy, and it is also right on the edge of the Middle St. Vrain Creek. Although we've narrowed the choices, keep in mind that all campsites are scattered among the spruce, pine, and aspen trees, and all have tent pads, parking, and fire areas.

Enter Peaceful Valley first, cross Middle St. Vrain Creek and site 7 is directly to the left. A right turn takes you into a nice, small loop that starts with our favorite site, 1; circles counterclockwise to 2, 3, 4, 5, and 6; and then deposits you back to site 7. Continue to site 8, which is usually the host site; site 9 is on the right, next to the drinking water. A cluster of sites— 10, 11, 12, 13, and 14—are on the left. Across from them is site 9, and next to that is site 15. Site 16 is also on this right side and site 17 is the last on the left. Sites 8 through 17 should actually receive high honorable mention since these sites have the dense trees and have more shelter than sites 1 through 7.

Leave Peaceful Valley and enter into Camp Dick. On the right are sites 1 through 9, which are quite close together and have few trees or little privacy. However, favorite sites 40 and 41 are on the left and are very different with tons of privacy and beautiful scenery. Continue toward the right and pass sites 10 and 12, which are favorites; 11, 13, and 14 come next; and a small loop begins with favorites 15, 16, curves to an okay 17, and then comes back to two

ADDRESS:	Peaceful Valley and Camp Dick Boulder Ranger District 2140 Yarmouth Avenue Boulder, CO 80301
OPERATED BY:	USDA Forest Service, Arapaho and Roosevelt National Forests, Pawnee National Grassland
INFORMATION:	(303) 541-2500; www.fs.fed.us/r2/arnf
OPEN:	Mid-May– mid-October
SITES:	58 (Camp Dick, 41; Peaceful Valley, 17)
EACH SITE HAS:	Picnic table, fire rings, upright grills, tent pads
ASSIGNMENT:	By reservation
REGISTRATION:	By phone (877) 444-6777, online at www.reserveusa.com, or self-registration on site
FACILITIES:	Water, vault toilets
PARKING:	At campsite
FEE:	$14 per night, $17 for oversized sites, an additional $9 fee added to each Internet or phone reservation
ELEVATION:	8,650 feet
RESTRICTIONS:	*Pets:* On leash *Fires:* In designated areas *Alcohol:* Allowed *Vehicles:* 55 feet *Other:* 14-day stay limit; maximum 8–12 people per site, varies by site

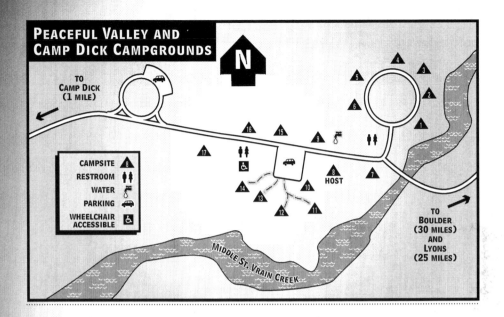

PEACEFUL VALLEY AND CAMP DICK CAMPGROUNDS

TO CAMP DICK (1 MILE)

CAMPSITE
RESTROOM
WATER
PARKING
WHEELCHAIR ACCESSIBLE

HOST

TO BOULDER (30 MILES) AND LYONS (25 MILES)

MIDDLE ST. VRAIN CREEK

GETTING THERE

Peaceful Valley Campground is off of CO 72 (also known as the Peak to Peak Highway) at mile-marker 50, approximately 19 miles north of Nederland and 20 miles south of Estes Park. It may also be accessed via CO 66 west to Lyons, then southwest on CO 7 for approximately 12 miles to CO 72, and south on CO 72, approximately 4 miles.

GPS COORDINATES

UTM Zone (WGS84) 13T
Easting   0456600
Northing   4442400
Latitude   N 40° 7' 57"
Longitude   W 105° 30' 32"

more favorites, 18 and 19. Sites 20, 21, 22, 23 are on the right side of a new loop; sites 24, 26, 28 are inside the loop and not recommended. Sites 26 and 27 are on the opposite side. Site 26 wasn't a favorite because it sits in the open, and site 27 is very close to the vault toilet. As the loop ends, a straightaway hosts ten honorable mention sites. On the right are sites 29 through 34, and on the left are sites 39 through 36. Site 35 is at the far end of all of these sites—so far at the end of the turnaround loop, in fact, that we really like it.

This area was once the site of a Civilian Conservation Corps camp established in the 1930s. Now, the campground is open to all and is normally full for the weekend by early Friday afternoon. So, plan to arrive early, consider making a reservation, and always try to take time off during the week to really take advantage of this beautiful place.

MAP

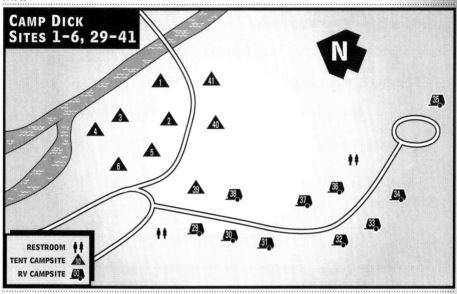

CAMP DICK
SITES 1–6, 29–41

N

RESTROOM
TENT CAMPSITE 00
RV CAMPSITE 00

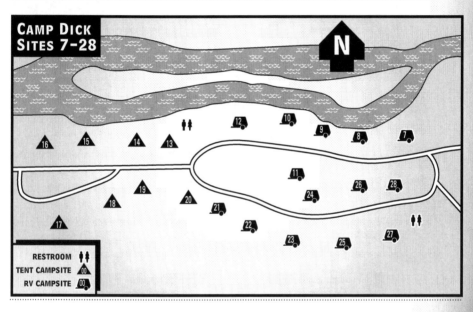

CAMP DICK
SITES 7–28

N

RESTROOM
TENT CAMPSITE 00
RV CAMPSITE 00

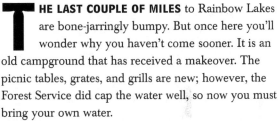

18
RAINBOW LAKES
CAMPGROUND

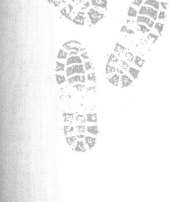

> *Rainbow Lakes is Boulder County's best high-country tent-camping getaway.*

THE LAST COUPLE OF MILES to Rainbow Lakes are bone-jarringly bumpy. But once here you'll wonder why you haven't come sooner. It is an old campground that has received a makeover. The picnic tables, grates, and grills are new; however, the Forest Service did cap the water well, so now you must bring your own water.

The campground is just south of Rocky Mountain National Park and is adjacent to the equally scenic Indian Peaks Wilderness. The forest here is upper-level montane, primarily lodgepole, with some Engelmann spruce and a few aspens struggling to survive. On my late June visit, the aspens had barely started leafing out. Their short growth time coincides with the short time this campground is open.

If you are in the area, stay here. The Rainbow Lakes are only half a mile from the campground. Make your visit up to the lakes for the day, and camp down at the campground. That preserves the natural resource and concentrates your impact at the campground. Rainbow Lakes Campground can also be a base camp for exploring the east side of Rocky Mountain National Park. Be forewarned: this campground receives heavy weekend use in the late summer.

Rainbow Lakes Campground lies along a stream emanating from the Rainbow Lakes that feed into Caribou Creek. Willows and beaver ponds break up the meadow to your left; on your right is a rising woodland. The first three sites are on a spur to your right. One is a pull-through site, but don't expect to find RVers up here unless they enjoy tearing up their rig. Continue up the main drive and another loop spurs off your right. It contains six campsites that are beneath conifers. The two sites inside the spur loop are a little small.

The rest of the campsites border the stream and are spread apart well beneath the trees. The last campsite is

RATINGS

Beauty: ☆ ☆ ☆ ☆
Privacy: ☆ ☆ ☆
Spaciousness: ☆ ☆ ☆ ☆
Quiet: ☆ ☆ ☆ ☆
Security: ☆ ☆ ☆
Cleanliness: ☆ ☆ ☆

away from the others, next to the trailhead parking area for Rainbow Lakes. Three vault toilets for this small campground are overkill, but at least you won't have to walk far to the bathroom no matter where you are camped.

Stated simply, come here during the week or Sunday night if at all possible. Not only is the campground full on weekends but there is also significant traffic coming through the campground to and from the Rainbow Lakes trailhead.

From Nederland you drove part of the Peak to Peak Scenic Byway. Continue to enjoy this drive north to Estes Park, where there are supplies, and south to Black Hawk and Central City, where there is legalized gambling. The casinos offer limited stakes gaming.

However, a sure bet is the Indian Peaks Wilderness next door. The glaciers in the Indian Peaks are the southernmost ones in North America. This high wilderness starts at 10,700 feet. Much of the scenery is austere tundra, rock, and ice. The Rainbow Lakes Trail goes the half mile to the lakes and is a must-hike.

The Arapaho Glacier Trail runs in and out of the wilderness a few miles up to the Arapaho Glacier overlook. The glacier is on this side of North Arapaho Peak. It is 6 miles from the trailhead to the Arapaho Pass Trail. Other trailheads into the busy Indian Peaks lie north off forest roads that intersect the Peak to Peak Byway.

Another area to consider is the Wild Basin of Rocky Mountain National Park. This is a watery place, where many cascades tumble down from the heights and picturesque lakes lie beneath craggy peaks. The basin is north on the Peak to Peak Byway. Get hiking information from the Ranger Station there.

For a little bit of interesting civilization, try the college town of Boulder 45 minutes down Boulder Canyon. This eclectic place is known for its diversity and beauty. Take a walk down Pearl Street, where the streets are blocked off and the dining, shopping, and culture reigns supreme. Nearby Nederland, albeit a more toned down version of Boulder, earns honorable mention with their few, but quality restaurants and a great grocery store. Make a visit to Nederland part of your Rainbow Lakes experience.

KEY INFORMATION

ADDRESS: Rainbow Lakes Campground Boulder Ranger District 2140 Yarmouth Avenue Boulder, CO 80301

OPERATED BY: USDA Forest Service, Arapaho and Roosevelt National Forests, Pawnee National Grassland

INFORMATION: (303) 541-2500; www.fs.fed.us/r2/arnf

OPEN: July–September, sometimes longer

SITES: 16

EACH SITE HAS: Picnic table, tent pad, fire grate, stand-up grill

ASSIGNMENT: First come, first served; no reservation

REGISTRATION: Self-registration on-site

FACILITIES: Vault toilets (bring water)

PARKING: At campsites only

FEE: $8 per night, plus $3 for a second vehicle

ELEVATION: 10,000 feet

RESTRICTIONS: *Pets:* On leash only
Fires: In fire grates only
Alcohol: At campsites only
Vehicles: 20-feet
Other: 14-day stay limit; maximum 8 people allowed per site

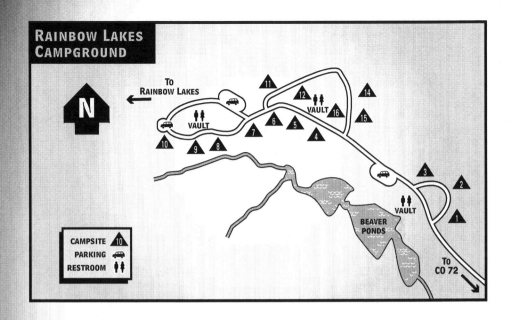

GETTING THERE

From Nederland, drive north on CO 72 for 6.5 miles to FS 298 (also known as CR 116). There will be a sign for University of Colorado Mountain Research Station. Turn left on FS 298 and follow it for 6 miles to Rainbow Lakes Campground.

GPS COORDINATES

UTM Zone (WGS84)   13T
Easting   0451180
Northing   4429090
Latitude   N 40° 0' 37.5"
Longitude   W 105° 34' 16"

ROBBERS **R**OOST CONJURES UP IMAGES of wild-West outlaws and hideouts for bandits that may have just had a shootout at the OK Corral. True to its name, this campground offers plenty of sites to escape to in its dark, wooded terrain and remote location. At the base of Berthoud Pass, far from the buzzing of the I-70 corridor, modern outlaws can find peace and hide out from a nagging boss or mounting bills. Never far from modern comforts, campers at Robbers Roost may also step out and hit the small mountain town of Winter Park if a cold one will hit the spot.

Robbers Roost is a spread-out campground in the tall timber at the western base of Berthoud Pass. RVs are not officially banned here, but the parking spots are smaller than most and many sites simply can not host a large rig. Robbers Roost is a tried-and-true Colorado mountain campground with a traditional "gather around the campfire in the pines" atmosphere. The dispersed arrangement is perfect for naturalists who don't like a strict layout or cookie-cutter feel at each campsite. The terrain allows for little room at each site and is suitable for small and midsized tents only. Level areas for tents are not in abundance, and it takes some time at each site to scope for the best place to lay your tarp— a refreshing change from the perfectly lined up tent pads at some campgrounds.

Entering the campground and starting a counter-clockwise loop, the road is visible from site 1, but sites 2 through 6, at the beginning of the campground immediately eliminate the view of the highway. These five sites are the best in the campground because they are private and spacious. Sites 2 and 3 are best for space and flatness, while site 6 is the favorite because it is more private and at the end of a loop. A small stream passes these five sites and site 6 even has a small footbridge

> *A campground escape that is worthy of the outlaw in all of us.*

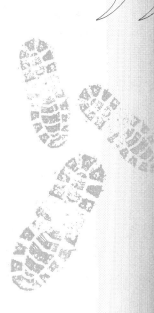

RATINGS

Beauty: ✿ ✿ ✿ ✿
Privacy: ✿ ✿ ✿ ✿
Spaciousness: ✿ ✿ ✿ ✿
Quiet: ✿ ✿ ✿
Security: ✿ ✿ ✿
Cleanliness: ✿ ✿ ✿ ✿

ADDRESS: Robbers Roost
Sulphur Ranger
District
9 Ten Mile Drive,
P.O. Box 10
Granby, CO 80446

OPERATED BY: Fraser River Valley
Lions Club under an
agreement
with USDA Forest
Service, Arapaho,
and Roosevelt
National Forests,
Pawnee National
Grassland

INFORMATION: (970) 887-4100

OPEN: Memorial Day–
Labor Day; may
open later in heavy
snow years

SITES: 11

EACH SITE HAS: Fire grate or fire pit,
picnic table

ASSIGNMENT: First come, first
served

REGISTRATION: On site

FACILITIES: Vault toilets,
no water

PARKING: 1 space at each
campsite

FEE: $12

ELEVATION: 9,826 feet

RESTRICTIONS: *Pets:* On leash
Fires: In designated
areas
Alcohol: Allowed
Vehicles: 25 feet
Other: 14-day stay
limit, 5 people
per site with a
maximum of 2 tents
per site

you cross for campsite access. Site 8 offers less privacy since it's in the middle of the loop. Sites 7, 9, 10, and 11 are on the opposite side and uphill of the loop and are okay, but tent space is smallest at these.

Robbers Roost does get a little road noise from US 40, but this is a mountain pass, not a major inter-state. This area also receives a huge amount of snow accumulation and typically opens later than the sched-uled Memorial Day.

Winter Park and Mary Jane ski areas are just down the road and offer fun all year, like mountain biking and hiking in the summer and camping season. The nearby Moffat Road is an abandoned high alpine railroad grade, now a dirt road open to cars and bikes. Moffat Road is a fun, lung-buster of a mountain-bike ride up to Rollins Pass, and a great cruiser of a ride down. The town of Winter Park is only ten minutes away from the campground and is a great place to eat, shop, and even catch a movie.

The Sulphur Ranger District, composed of more than 400,000 acres in Grand County, Colorado, is sur-rounded by mountains, meadows, and lakes. To the west of Robbers Roost, the three lakes of Grand, Granby, and Shadow Mountain are fun for the day with a small boat or fishing pole. The Stillwater area next to Grand Lake has miles of trails for four-wheel-drive enthusiasts.

To the east of Robbers Roost, the ski area on top of Berthoud Pass is permanently closed, but the region offers tons of hiking and access to plenty of wildlife and wildflowers.

The 12,000 to 13,000 foot mountains above the campground make up the spine of the Continental Divide. The tiny Fraser River that starts in the valley, near Robbers Roost, grows to become the massive Colorado River and flows into the Pacific Ocean to the west.

In contrast, and in the magical allure of the Continental Divide, all precipitation on the other side of the ridge above the campground ends up in tributaries that feed into the Atlantic Ocean to the east. Avalanche shoots on this side of Berthoud Pass are always awe inspiring, fun to locate, and less threatening during the summer camping season.

MAP

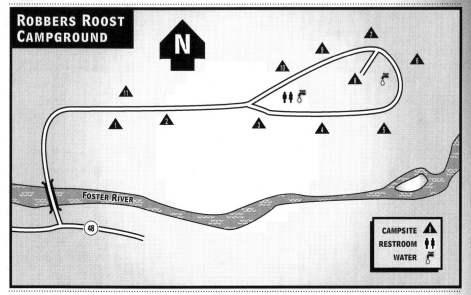

ROBBERS ROOST
CAMPGROUND

FOSTER RIVER

48

CAMPSITE
RESTROOM
WATER

GETTING THERE

Travel 5 miles south of
Winter Park ski area on
US 40 to the base of
Berthoud Pass.

GPS COORDINATES

UTM Zone (WGS84) 13S
Easting 0436640
Northing 4406260
Latitude N 39° 48' 21"
Longitude W 105° 44' 23"

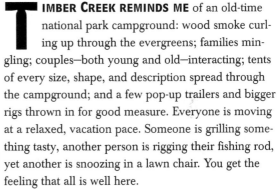

> *Timber Creek is your best bet for getting a good tent campsite in Rocky Mountain National Park.*

TIMBER **C**REEK **REMINDS ME** of an old-time national park campground: wood smoke curling up through the evergreens; families mingling; couples—both young and old—interacting; tents of every size, shape, and description spread through the campground; and a few pop-up trailers and bigger rigs thrown in for good measure. Everyone is moving at a relaxed, vacation pace. Someone is grilling something tasty, another person is rigging their fishing rod, yet another is snoozing in a lawn chair. You get the feeling that all is well here.

Timber Creek lies in a wooded flat alongside the headwaters of the Colorado River. Trail Ridge Road forms the other boundary. Lodgepole pine is the primary tree here. Pine needles and an occasional rock form the understory. The campsites are spread out in this sizable campground on a main drive with four loops spurring off it. The odd thing is that the loops are named after trees that don't even grow in this park (dogwood is one example)! The main drive passes the Ranger Station and passes some large campsites. Just across from the Ranger Station are the first tent-only campsites. The tent campsites have a car pull-in area, then your campsite is in the woods across planted wood poles separating the camping and parking areas.

The main drive swings alongside the willows of the Colorado River. A few riverside sites are in mixed shade and sun and are the best campsites here. The river and mountain views are nice. The rest of the campground is well shaded by lodgepole pine. The first camping loop splits off to the left and has tent-only and general-use sites. The next loop has tent-only and general-use campsites, also. The third loop has only general campsites, but tenters are the majority here too. The fourth and final loop has mostly tent-only sites.

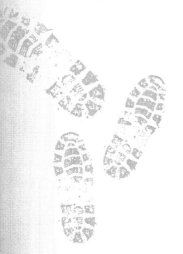

RATINGS

Beauty: ✿ ✿ ✿ ✿
Privacy: ✿ ✿ ✿
Spaciousness: ✿ ✿ ✿
Quiet: ✿ ✿ ✿
Security: ✿ ✿ ✿ ✿ ✿
Cleanliness: ✿ ✿ ✿ ✿

There are several beaver ponds off in the meadow toward the river. Other wildlife, notably moose and elk, have been known to wander through the campground. (I saw some elk during my visit here.)

Water spigots and comfort stations are spread throughout Rocky Mountain National Park's least busy campground. However, it often fills during the peak season. Timber Creek nears capacity nearly every night from late June to early August. You can generally find a campsite until late in the day Sunday through Thursday. Campsites are usually gone by noon on Friday and Saturday. Finding a campsite in the off-season is no problem, though campground roads are not snowplowed.

If you haven't driven Trail Ridge Road, drive it. It is a rite of passage for first-time park visitors. Campers also like to see the wildlife, fish, and hike the area trails. The Never Summer Ranch Trail leaves from the lower part of the campground. It is a mere half-a-mile walk to this early-era guest ranch. The buildings and grounds have been preserved by the park. Interpretive rangers are on site there in the summer.

The Green Mountain Loop is a popular day hike for Timber Creek campers. It starts down US 34. See Big Meadow and the ruins of a pioneer cabin on this 8-mile tramp. The much shorter River Trail Loop starts down by the Kawuneeche Visitor Center. It runs along the Colorado River and offers views of the Never Summer Mountains above. The path to Timber Lake presents good scenery and is a 10-mile round-trip hike. There are many other trails in the area. The ranger on duty at the campground can steer you on a hike to meet your abilities and desires.

The Colorado River offers fair fishing for brook, brown, rainbow, and cutthroat trout. But serious fishers will head down to the Arapaho National Recreation Area by Grand Lake. The fish are bigger, and the lake is stocked regularly.

Back at the campground, ranger programs are held every night during the summer from mid-June to Labor Day. But mostly campers at Timber Creek will be seen piddling around their campsites. It's called relaxing and having a good time.

KEY INFORMATION

ADDRESS: Timber Creek Campground Rocky Mountain National Park Estes Park, CO 80517

OPERATED BY: National Park Service; Rocky Mountain National Park

INFORMATION: (970) 586-1206; www.nps.gov/romo

OPEN: All year

SITES: 33 tent-only sites, 67 other

EACH SITE HAS: Picnic table, fire grate, tent pad

ASSIGNMENT: First come, first served; no reservation

REGISTRATION: Self-registration on site

FACILITIES: Water spigot, flush toilets, phone (no water late September–May)

PARKING: At campsites only

FEE: $20 per night, $14 in off season (when water is turned off), a separate park entrance fee applies

ELEVATION: 8,900 feet

RESTRICTIONS: *Pets:* On leash only *Fires:* In fire grates only *Alcohol:* At campsites only *Vehicles:* 38 feet *Other:* 7-day stay limit per campsite

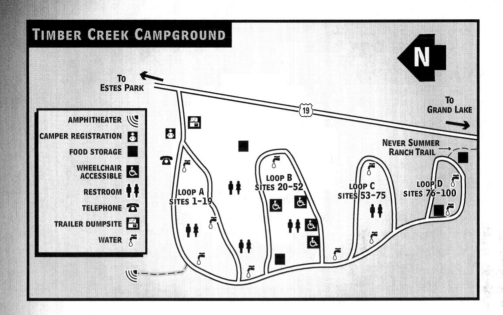

GETTING THERE

From Grand Lake, head north on US 34 for 10 miles and Timber Creek Campground will be on your left.

GPS COORDINATES

UTM Zone (WGS84)   13T
Easting   0427720
Northing   4470200
Latitude   N 40° 22' 44.9"
Longitude   W 105° 51' 5.6"

21
WESTON PASS CAMPGROUND

NAMED AFTER THE SCENIC BREAK in the Mosquito Range, Weston Pass is an often-bypassed campground adjacent to an often-bypassed wilderness. I wonder why, since the neatness, cleanliness, and lack of overuse of the campground were evident immediately upon arrival. One look at the mountains of the Buffalo Peaks Wilderness will make you wonder why you didn't get here sooner. The answer lies partly in what surrounds the area—several other, more popular wildernesses and campgrounds lie between the Buffalo Peaks and the major metropolitan areas of the state.

I prefer smaller campgrounds; they are usually a little more out of the way (read: fewer big rigs) and seem to bring out the neighborliness in your fellow tent campers. Weston Pass has only 14 campsites in an area that I've seen fit twice that many at other campgrounds. The campsites are large and spaced very far apart beneath a forest of lodgepole pine that is supported by other evergreens and a few straggling aspen. The ground cover is mostly smaller trees and assorted rocks and boulders. Landscaping timbers and short concrete posts have been tastefully laid out to keep cars and camping areas distinct. This is part of what gives Weston Pass a certain orderliness not always found at other Forest Service campgrounds.

The South Fork of the South Platte River and a low ridge dividing this creek from Rich Creek surround the campground. Head along the main drive and admire the size of the campsites set back in the woods several feet from their respective parking areas. Notice the Ridgeview Trail splitting off between two campsites. The seven sites on the main drive give way to a loop road that swings near the South Fork. The loop offers secluded campsites that drop down toward the clearly audible creek. As the loop swings around,

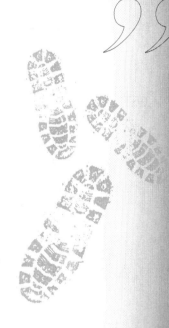

> *Weston Pass is one of the nicer Forest Service campgrounds in Colorado.*

RATINGS

Beauty: ✿ ✿ ✿
Privacy: ✿ ✿ ✿ ✿
Spaciousness: ✿ ✿ ✿ ✿
Quiet: ✿ ✿ ✿ ✿
Security: ✿ ✿ ✿
Cleanliness: ✿ ✿ ✿ ✿ ✿

ADDRESS:	Weston Pass Campground South Park Ranger District 320 US 285 Fairplay, CO 80440
OPERATED BY:	USDA Forest Service, Pike and San Isabel National Forests, Cimarron and Comanche National Grasslands
INFORMATION:	(719) 836-2031; www.fs.fed.us/r2/ psicc/sopa
OPEN:	May–September
SITES:	14
EACH SITE HAS:	Picnic table, fire grate
ASSIGNMENT:	First come, first served; no reservation
REGISTRATION:	Self-registration on site
FACILITIES:	Hand-pump well, vault toilets
PARKING:	At campsites only
FEE:	$10 per night
ELEVATION:	10,200 feet
RESTRICTIONS:	*Pets:* On leash only *Fires:* In fire grates only *Alcohol:* At campsites only *Vehicles:* 25 feet *Other:* 14-day stay limit

one campsite, 11, is actually a walk-in tent site farther up the creek, away from everyone else. A few more of those large campsites are banked against the low, rocky ridge that shades the campground in the late afternoon.

The well is out by the main road just before you bridge the South Fork. Two vault toilets conveniently serve Weston Pass. This quiet campground rarely fills, except on holidays, when you should be avoiding campgrounds anyway.

For your evening leg-stretcher, take the Ridgeview Trail 1 mile to an overlook on the point between the drainages of Rich Creek and South Fork. Take note that this trail also connects you to the Rich Creek Trail, which dives into the heart of the Buffalo Peaks Wilderness. The forests here, from piñon-juniper on the lower western slopes to the bristlecone pines of the highlands, are thick with both trees and wildlife, from bighorn sheep to beaver. This area is decidedly lacking in the human species compared to other wildernesses this close to Denver and Colorado Springs.

One of the better day hikes in the Pike National Forest takes off near Weston Pass Campground. Make an 11-mile loop taking the Rich Creek Trail up to Buffalo Meadows and picking up the Rough and Tumbling Trail back down. The Buffalo Peaks Wilderness is also an excellent place to build up your peak-bagging skills. Though they are not fourteeners, East and West Buffalo Peak exceed 13,000 feet and have definite tree lines that you pass on the way to sizable rock faces to scale with little difficulty. Take the Rough and Tumbling Trail beyond Buffalo Meadows to the headwaters of Rough and Tumbling Creek, then ascend to the pass where the Rough and Tumbling Trail starts to descend. Veer east first to West Buffalo Peak then East Buffalo Peak. Return to the Rough and Tumbling Trail and backtrack to the campground. This makes a very long day hike, so leave early in the morning for this adventure.

If you don't feel like walking to a view, make the drive up to 11,921-foot Weston Pass. Here, you can look north at a seemingly endless range of peaks. You can also stay down low and fish your way around the

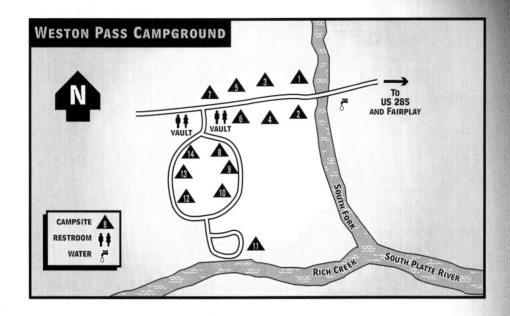

South Fork or other waters in the wilderness. Or you can enjoy the subtle, relaxing beauty of the Weston Pass Campground. Pass those other places by for a chance to enjoy the Weston Pass area.

GETTING THERE

From the Ranger Station in Fairplay, drive south on US 285 for 5 miles to CR 5 (Weston Pass Road). Continue on CR 5 until it merges with CR 22 at 7 miles. The campground will be on your left 4 miles ahead on CR 22.

GPS COORDINATES

UTM Zone (WGS84)	13S
Easting	0402280
Northing	4325390
Latitude	N 39° 4' 19.9"
Longitude	W 106° 7' 47"

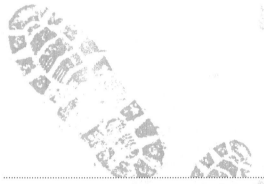

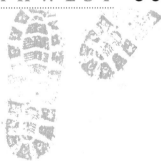

NORTHWEST COLORADO

22
BIG DOMINGUEZ CAMPGROUND

LET'S SEE . . . **MOUNTAIN BIKING,** canyon hiking, canyon hiking, trout fishing, scenic drives, Indian petroglyphs, mining ghost towns, canoeing the Gunnison River . . . all accessible from a free campground made for tent campers that happens to be one of the best in the state. This is Dominguez Canyon. Bureau of Land Management (BLM) campgrounds are generally less known to the public than national-park and national-forest campgrounds. Once you find this little gem, you will be making return trips.

Drop off the Uncompahgre Plateau a bit and descend into Dominguez Canyon. Deep red cliffs are behind you. Below you, bordering Big Dominguez Creek, is a dense forest of large cottonwoods, complemented by thickets of willow and alder, making for a very green scene. Across the canyon, sage gives way to ponderosa pine and Douglas fir intermingling with piñon and juniper.

The air cools down as you approach the clear, chattering creek. Off to your right is a fenced-in grassy area below the cottonwoods. On the far side of a wood fence, three picnic tables lie along the cool waters and offer creekside picnicking. The deep shade and the chilled air along the creek makes a great escape from the heat of the summer sun in the Colorado River Valley. Farther on, just across the shallow ford of Big Dominguez Creek, lies a single site in the very thick of the cottonwoods. This campsite is for privacy lovers.

Just upstream from this secluded campsite is a small footbridge connecting both sides of the campground. The entrance road fords the creek and to your right is a small meadow and parking area. An attractive log fence guards more campsites. The cottonwoods here are smaller, still providing ample shade, but letting campers enjoy the views around them. Small openings in the fence allow campers to access

> *Enjoy both the red canyons and green forests of the Uncompahgre Plateau from Dominguez.*

RATINGS

Beauty: ✩ ✩ ✩ ✩
Privacy: ✩ ✩ ✩
Spaciousness: ✩ ✩ ✩ ✩
Quiet: ✩ ✩ ✩ ✩
Security: ✩ ✩ ✩
Cleanliness: ✩ ✩ ✩

ADDRESS: Big Dominguez
Campground
2815 H Road
Grand Junction, CO
81506

OPERATED BY: Bureau of Land
Management

INFORMATION: (970) 244-3000;
www.co.blm.gov/
gjra/dominguezcg
.htm

OPEN: Mid-May–
mid-October

SITES: 9

EACH SITE HAS: Picnic table, fire ring

ASSIGNMENT: First come,
first served; no
reservation

REGISTRATION: No registration

FACILITIES: Vault toilets
(no water)

PARKING: At tent camping
parking areas

FEE: None

ELEVATION: 7,500 feet

RESTRICTIONS: *Pets:* On leash only
Fires: In fire rings
only
Alcohol: At campsites
only
Vehicles: None
Other: 14-day stay
limit

sites on the far side, which allows for tent-only camping. The brush rises high enough to make for good campsite privacy.

Three of the first five campsites have two picnic tables each, allowing for larger parties. One campsite is far back in the woods and looks over a mesa that comes to a point above Big Dominguez Creek and an unnamed tributary.

Two other parties joined me on my stay. The small campground rarely fills, so make your plans and come on up. There is no water provided, though springwater from a pipe is located on the entrance road just above the campground. You could also use the water from Big Dominguez Creek and treat it. Two new vault toilets have been put in on both sides of the creek.

The campground is perched on the edge of the 70,000-acre Big Dominguez Wilderness Study Area. The BLM expects this area ultimately to become a full-fledged wilderness. One look and you'll agree that it should be preserved.

A good way to get that look is on the Big Dominguez Trail, which starts at the campground. You can head down the canyon and enumerate reasons for preservation. On the lower part of the canyon are Indian petroglyphs; the best way to access the cliff drawings is from Cactus Park. Watch for the sign for Cactus Park on Colorado 141 as you head for the campground, then take the trail toward Triangle Mesa and take the right split down to the Big Dominguez Creek and the petroglyphs. You can also follow the Smith Point Trail up Dominguez Canyon from the campground.

If you like fishing small creeks for trout as much as I do, you'll love Big Dominguez Creek. Take the Big Dominguez Trail down the canyon and simply drop into the creek drainage, then work your way up— secretively I might add—and cast with small spinners. Rainbow trout will positively attack your lure. If you want to ride in the water instead of walking through it, check with outfitters in Whitewater and Grand Junction. The nearby Gunnison River offers some decent canoeing that is more of a relaxed float than a hair-raising whitewater ride.

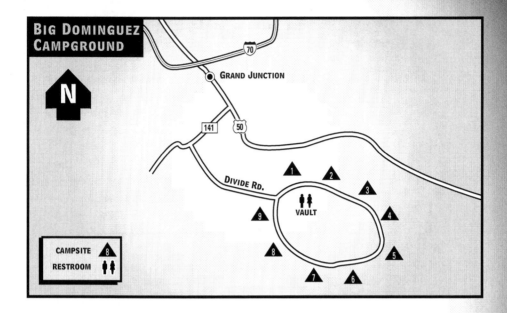

Mountain bikers take note that the heart of the 140-mile Tabeguache Trail passes right through this campground. You can take the trail up to the plateau or drop down toward Cactus Park. Send for a map of the Tabeguache Trail from the BLM office in Grand Junction.

Auto tourists will want to return to CO 141 and drive farther up Unaweep Canyon toward Gateway. In the mountains east of Gateway, many old mining sites and miners' shacks are on BLM lands. Again, inquire at the BLM office for details; you'll like what they have to offer in this part of the state.

GETTING THERE

From Grand Junction, drive southeast on US 50 for 10 miles to CO 141 and the town of Whitewater. Turn right on CO 141 and follow it for 11.5 miles to Divide Road. Turn left on Divide Road and follow it for 5 miles to a fork in the road. Turn left at the fork. There is a sign and arrow saying "Big Dominguez Resource Conservation Area."

Follow this road 5 miles to Big Dominguez Campground.

GPS COORDINATES

UTM Zone (WGS84)   12S
Easting   0711890
Northing   4291590
Latitude   N 38° 44' 51.9"
Longitude   W 108° 33' 41"

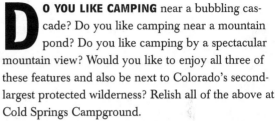

> *Cold Springs is both the grandstand and springboard for enjoying the eastern Flat Tops Wilderness.*

DO YOU LIKE CAMPING near a bubbling cascade? Do you like camping near a mountain pond? Do you like camping by a spectacular mountain view? Would you like to enjoy all three of these features and also be next to Colorado's second-largest protected wilderness? Relish all of the above at Cold Springs Campground.

Now, this place isn't perfect, but Cold Springs is an earthly delight. Here, you can leave your tent, fish and hike all day, then return to your little scenic mountain heaven.

All right, let's get to the bad part. It is a little closer to the road than is truly ideal. The campsites could stand to be a little more level. The campground as a whole is pretty broken in, but other than that, it's great.

Turn into the short campground drive and pass the first campsite on your left, in an open meadow with the best of alpine views. Snow-covered Flat Top Mountain lies across the Bear River, which rushes from Stillwater Reservoir above. Behind you, tree-covered slopes rise to mountain lakes. There is a good view down the valley of Bear River as well.

Cross over a small stream, then enter the small loop road. To your right is the mountain pond. Above it, on the hill, are two other streams noisily dropping over rocks into the pond. The second campsite lies in an open meadow next to the pond and the first stream. This is the largest and most popular campsite. The third campsite is close to the pond as well. It offers all views, but no shade.

The fourth campsite is closest to the cascades and has some shade-providing spruce. The fifth campsite is set off in a forested corner of the campground beside a stream of its own. This is the shadiest and most private campsite. An outhouse lies in the center of the loop

RATINGS

Beauty: ✩ ✩ ✩ ✩
Privacy: ✩ ✩
Spaciousness: ✩ ✩ ✩
Quiet: ✩ ✩ ✩
Security: ✩ ✩ ✩
Cleanliness: ✩ ✩ ✩ ✩

and a water spigot is close to all campers in this small campground.

If Cold Springs is full—with only five sites it may very well be on summer weekends—try Horseshoe Campground just a little way back down Bear River Road. It is has seven campsites and is more forested than Cold Springs; consequently it doesn't have the inspiring views. Cold Springs offers car-free access to the recreational opportunities of the Bear River corridor.

The Flat Tops Wilderness is all around you: cliffs towering over alpine tundra and subalpine terrain, where spruce–fir forests give way to more than 110 fish-filled lakes and ponds. Another 100 miles of streams flow through this angler's fantasyland. Just a five-minute jaunt up the road from Cold Springs is a major trailhead, Stillwater, leading into the Flat Tops.

To survey your kingdom for a day, take the North Derby Trail, #1122. Cross the Stillwater Dam to a large park, then climb into the wooded highlands through a burned area, coming to an 11,200-foot pass after about two miles.

Turn left at the pass, leaving the maintained trail, and stay on the divide, rising to the peak of Flat Top Mountain at mile 4. There is a rock pile at the 12,354-foot summit. Look down and see if you can see your friends or spot your tent back at the campsite. You can also stay on the maintained trail and come to Hooper and Keepner Lakes at 3 miles. These are great fishing lakes.

The Bear River Trail, #1120, leaves Stillwater Reservoir and goes west into the wilderness. Pass Mosquito Lake at mile 1.5, a scenic, yet dubious, destination, then climb toward the high country. Once up high, you can go along the Flat Tops in either direction or drop down toward Trappers Lake. The high-country trails are fairly level, for scenic, mild hiking.

The East Fork Trail, #1119, splits off the Bear River Trail and heads north into some superb vistas. Pass Little Causeway Lake at mile 1.2, then climb up toward the Devils Causeway, a side destination from the East Fork Trail. This is a narrow stretch (4 feet wide) of the Flat Top plateau that drops 1,500 feet in

KEY INFORMATION

ADDRESS: Cold Springs Campground Yampa Ranger District P.O. Box 7, 300 Roselawn Avenue Yampa, CO 80483

OPERATED BY: USDA Forest Service, Medicine Bow–Routt National Forests, Thunder Basin National Grassland

INFORMATION: (970) 638-4516; www.fs.fed.us/r2/mbr

OPEN: Memorial Day–September 30

SITES: 5

EACH SITE HAS: Picnic table, fire grate

ASSIGNMENT: First come, first served; no reservation

REGISTRATION: Self-registration on site

FACILITIES: Water spigot, vault toilets, trash collection

PARKING: At campsites only

FEE: $10 per night

ELEVATION: 10,200 feet

RESTRICTIONS: *Pets:* On leash only
Fires: In fire grates only
Alcohol: At campsites only
Vehicles: 22 feet
Other: 14-day stay limit

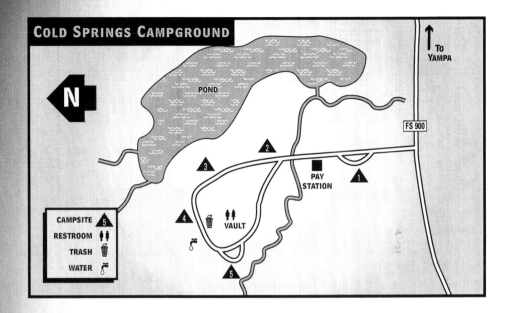

COLD SPRINGS CAMPGROUND

To YAMPA

POND

FS 900

PAY STATION

VAULT

CAMPSITE
RESTROOM
TRASH
WATER

GETTING THERE

From Yampa, drive southwest on CR 7 for 17 miles as it turns into FS 900.
Proceed on FS 900 for about 10 miles. Cold Springs will be on your right.

either direction. On the main trail you will come to many small lakes and, finally, Causeway Lake at 5 miles. Anglers, be sure to bring your rods.

For those who want hike-free fishing, there are three reservoirs for fishing in the Bear River Corridor. The closest is Stillwater; Yampa and Yamcola reservoirs are downstream. In between these reservoirs flows the Bear River. Anglers can be seen bank-fishing the lakes and walking the meadows of Bear River. All these waters are stocked.

Limited supplies can be bought back down in Yampa. When you come to Cold Springs, expect to be busy—the great view at the campground will inspire you to be a part of the scenery.

GPS COORDINATES

UTM Zone (WGS84)   13T
Easting   0318680
Northing   4432940
Latitude   N 40° 1' 38.3"
Longitude   W 107° 7' 29"

24
COLORADO NATIONAL MONUMENT: SADDLEHORN CAMPGROUND

SOME FOLKS JUST GO FOR IT when they see something. In 1907, Jim Otto came to the canyon country southwest of Grand Junction and deemed it the most beautiful place he had ever seen. He thought it worthy to be a national park; he developed trails single-handedly among the forests and rock sculptures while simultaneously promoting the land with a few converts from Grand Junction. Four years later, Colorado National Monument was established. Jim's devotion to the park persisted until 1927, when he relinquished his $1-per-month job as park caretaker.

What foresight he had in protecting such a colorful landscape! Now, you can enjoy it too. Saddlehorn Campground is near many park features and hosts a few features of its own. After climbing out of the valley below, veer left around the Saddlehorn (it really does look like the horn of a saddle) and enter the campground. A forest of juniper and piñon emerge from the rust-red soil. Occasional rocks emerge from the fiery dirt among the sage. The whole campground has a slight slope toward the cliffs of the Colorado Plateau, which drop off into the Grand Valley of the Colorado River. Across the valley are the East Tavaputs Plateau and the Grand Mesa. The views are striking.

The campground water spigots are tastefully piped into native stone that add a little extra touch to Saddlehorn. The junipers here are bushy; they provide decent campsite privacy, but the noonday sun will beat you down in midsummer. Be forewarned, from mid-May until early July, small gnats rule this area and can drive you buggy.

A Loop has 20 sites that offer great views into the valley. Several of the sites are screened from the loop road. B Loop is very similar to A Loop and has some very private sites and great views. The lights of Grand Junction shine down below after dark.

> *Deep canyons, red rock, and natural stone sculptures characterize this unique Colorado spectacle.*

RATINGS

Beauty: ✿ ✿ ✿
Privacy: ✿ ✿ ✿
Spaciousness: ✿ ✿ ✿
Quiet: ✿ ✿ ✿ ✿
Security: ✿ ✿ ✿ ✿
Cleanliness: ✿ ✿ ✿ ✿

KEY INFORMATION

ADDRESS: Colorado National Monument: Saddlehorn Campground Fruita, CO 81521

OPERATED BY: National Park Service

INFORMATION: (970) 858-3617; www.nps.gov/colm

OPEN: A Loop all year, B Loop April–mid-October, C Loop when necessary; no water in winter

SITES: 80

EACH SITE HAS: Picnic table, stand-up grill

ASSIGNMENT: First come, first served; no reservation

REGISTRATION: Self-registration on site

FACILITIES: Water spigots, flush toilets

PARKING: At campsites only

FEE: $10 per night

ELEVATION: 5,800 feet

RESTRICTIONS: *Pets:* On leash only
Fires: No wood fires, charcoal fires in grills only
Alcohol: At campsites only
Vehicles: None
Other: 14-day stay limit

C Loop is part of the original campground built in the 1930s. The campsites are a little smaller than what we are accustomed to today. It offers views of the valley and into the monument, but C Loop is only open if the other loops are full, which normally occurs during Memorial Day weekend only. Otherwise you can bank on getting a campsite here.

The best time to visit Colorado National Monument, on the advice of a long-time park ranger, is mid-September to mid-November. The weather has cooled, the bugs are long gone, and the hiking is great. You can actually walk from your tent to some of the best day hikes in the park. The Window Rock Trail makes a short loop and offers photographic views. The Canyon Rim Trail travels on the edge of Wedding Canyon for more views. And views are what this monument is all about. Springtime attracts locals for wildflower viewing.

Another ranger recommendation is the Ottos Trail. It drops down toward the Pipe Organ and overlooks the depths of Monument Canyon. If you are here during the summer, use the middle of the day to make the 23-mile scenic drive from one end of the park to the other. There are numerous overlooks—you will wear your brakes out stopping at all the dramatic canyon scenes. Road bikers also enjoy pedaling the scenic road. The combination of scenery against the backdrop of the plateau and valley country makes for one photo op after another!

There are several longer trails that range from 6 to 8 miles. The Monument Canyon Trail enters the heart of the natural rock sculptures. Climbers can be seen scaling Independence Rock. If you are interested in climbing, stop at the park visitor center, where they have a book on climbing routes in the monument. Whether you climb or not, remember to be up high at dark—the sunsets and sunrises here are something to see. Rangers hold interpretive programs on summer weekends.

Colorado National Monument is a destination in its own right. But if you are traveling along I-70, don't just glance up and say you've seen this place. The scenery will surprise you while you look down at the folks who thought it wasn't worth their time.

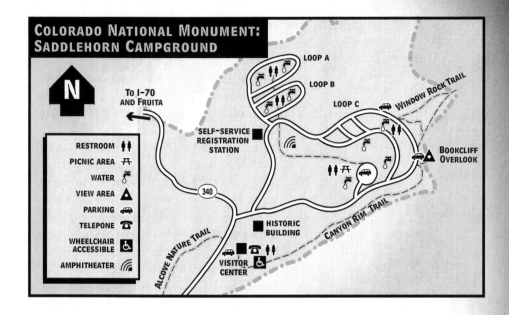

COLORADO NATIONAL MONUMENT: SADDLEHORN CAMPGROUND

N

To I-70 AND FRUITA

LOOP A
LOOP B
LOOP C

WINDOW ROCK TRAIL

SELF-SERVICE REGISTRATION STATION

BOOKCLIFF OVERLOOK

RESTROOM	👥
PICNIC AREA	🏕
WATER	🚰
VIEW AREA	△
PARKING	🚗
TELEPONE	☎
WHEELCHAIR ACCESSIBLE	♿
AMPHITHEATER	🎦

340

HISTORIC BUILDING

ALCOVE NATURE TRAIL

CANYON RIM TRAIL

VISITOR CENTER

GETTING THERE

From I-70 in Fruita, head south on CO 340 for 2 miles to the entrance of Colorado National Monument. Proceed into the monument for 5 miles, and Saddlehorn Campground will be on your left.

GPS COORDINATES

UTM Zone (WGS84)   12S
Easting   0702900
Northing   4322420
Latitude   N 39° 1'38.9"
Longitude   W 108° 39' 20"

DINOSAUR NATIONAL MONUMENT: ECHO PARK CAMPGROUND

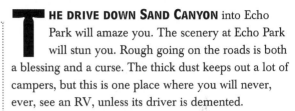

> *This is one of the best tent campgrounds in the entire national park system, but you might need an all-wheel-drive vehicle to reach it.*

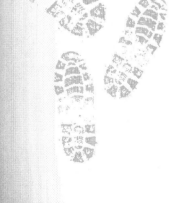

THE DRIVE DOWN **S**AND **C**ANYON into Echo Park will amaze you. The scenery at Echo Park will stun you. Rough going on the roads is both a blessing and a curse. The thick dust keeps out a lot of campers, but this is one place where you will never, ever, see an RV, unless its driver is demented.

Echo Park lies just below the confluence of the Green and Yampa Rivers. Colorful vertical canyon walls rise from across the river. The grassy meadow of Echo Park leads to another tan, gray, green, and black cliff face enclosing the park. Across the river is the stone sentinel of Steamboat Rock. A dense ribbon of box elder and cottonwood divides much of Echo Park from the river. The opening of Pool Creek Canyon narrows in the distance. More canyon walls and wooded mountains are downriver. The park continues upriver until the Yampa splits off to the right. Words can't begin to describe the true magnificence of Echo Park.

The campground is off to the left, between the river and the meadow as you enter Echo Park. The first campsite is riverside, all by itself; the river access and fee/information booth are past it. Next is a string of four campsites that look over the park from beneath dense, box elder trees. Small paths cut to the river from some of these campsites.

The dirt road continues, then more campsites appear on the riverbank. The picnic tables are lower than the parking spot for these sites. Farther down, the riparian woods break, allowing the next campsites to have views of the Green River and the sheer walls of the canyon beyond. An auto turnaround spot also serves as the parking area for the five walk-in tent campsites that extend upriver.

The first walk-in site sits alone beneath an old cottonwood. The others are a 150-yard walk to a grove of cottonwood and box elder trees that are not as dense

RATINGS

Beauty: ✪ ✪ ✪ ✪ ✪
Privacy: ✪ ✪ ✪ ✪
Spaciousness: ✪ ✪ ✪ ✪
Quiet: ✪ ✪ ✪ ✪ ✪
Security: ✪ ✪ ✪ ✪ ✪
Cleanliness: ✪ ✪ ✪ ✪

as the vehicle campsites. A water spigot and vault toilet serve these campsites. Other facilities are conveniently situated for all to use, even though the campground is strung over several hundred yards of the river.

You can count on getting a campsite during summer weekdays, but get to Echo Park early on summer weekends. Campsites are nearly always open during spring and fall. However, always call ahead to see if Echo Park is open, as rains can render the road impassable and close the campground.

On your way down Echo Park Road, enjoy the scenery of Sand and Pool canyons, then stop at the Chew Ranch. This site was not developed until the 1900s. The ranch was occupied as late as 1970, when the owner passed on. Other, more primitive ranch sites are also viewable. Next, you will come to a very interesting Indian petroglyph that was scratched high into the Sand Canyon wall. Whispering Cave is farther down. Walk close to it and feel the cool air on a summer day.

The Green River will lure you to its banks, but the swift current can make swimming hazardous. Fishing is negligible for channel catfish, which inhabit the stained waters. The photographic opportunities are numerous. You may also want to bring your camera on some day hikes that leave Echo Park.

The Sand Canyon Route heads up the Green River, then veers right up the Yampa to the first canyon on your right. You can follow the trail for miles up to Yampa Bench Road, but I recommend backtracking—it's less dusty than walking on the road. A good late-afternoon hike is the Mitten Park Route. It follows the Green River downstream, high above the left bank. Hike 1.5 miles to a grassy meadow, Mitten Park. It's another good place to look over Steamboat Rock.

Pats Draw is a quickie, canyon-sampler hike. Head back up the road out of the park and veer right just past the second creek ford. This is a short, but easy, there-and-back walk. You can also start back at the Chew Ranch, then follow the Pool Creek Route up the flow of Pool Creek, though the water course can dry up. It intersects Echo Park Road after 3 miles.

KEY INFORMATION

ADDRESS:	Dinosaur National Monument: Echo Park Campground 4545 East US 40 Dinosaur, CO 81610-9724
OPERATED BY:	National Park Service
INFORMATION:	(970) 374-3000 or (435) 781-7700; www.nps.gov/dino
OPEN:	May–September
SITES:	17
EACH SITE HAS:	Picnic table
ASSIGNMENT:	First come, first served; no reservation
REGISTRATION:	Self-registration on site
FACILITIES:	Water spigot, vault toilet
PARKING:	At campsites only
FEE:	$8 per night, one group site for $15 per night; park fee also required if you enter at the Dinosaur Quarry area on the Utah side of the park
ELEVATION:	5,000 feet
RESTRICTIONS:	*Pets:* On leash only *Fires:* No wood fires allowed, only charcoal fires in fire pans *Alcohol:* At campsites only *Vehicles:* No RVs or trailers; all-wheel-drive and high-clearance vehicles recommended *Other:* 14-day stay limit

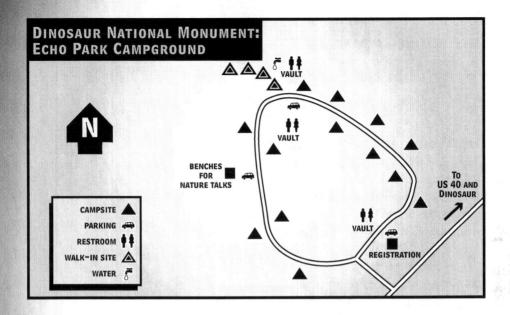

DINOSAUR NATIONAL MONUMENT: ECHO PARK CAMPGROUND

N

VAULT

VAULT

BENCHES FOR NATURE TALKS

To US 40 AND DINOSAUR

VAULT

REGISTRATION

CAMPSITE ▲
PARKING
RESTROOM
WALK-IN SITE △
WATER

GETTING THERE

From Dinosaur, head east on US 40 for 1.5 miles to the entrance for Dinosaur National Monument. Turn left on Harpers Corner Scenic Drive and follow it for 23 miles to Echo Park Road. Follow Echo Park Road for 8 dusty miles, then veer right at the signed turn for Echo Park. Follow this road for 5 miles to Echo Park Campground.

Dinosaur National Monument offers much outside of Echo Park. About 27 miles west of Dinosaur, Colorado, in the state of Utah, is the Dinosaur Quarry Visitor Center Museum that is overlaid on the fossilized bones of the dinosaurs that made this place a park. Unfortunately this museum, in Jensen, Utah, was closed indefinitely due to significant life, health, and safety issues. However, exhibits, film, fossil displays, ranger-led programs, and information are available in the outdoor visitor center near the park entrance in Jensen, Utah. Harpers Corner Scenic Drive offers a worthy auto tour. Some awe-inspiring views are at the end of day hikes that spur off the scenic drive. Commercial outfitters offer rafting opportunities into the deep canyons of the monument as well. It is impossible to resist telling your friends about this place.

GPS COORDINATES

UTM Zone (WGS84) 12T
Easting 0670790
Northing 4487980
Latitude N 40° 31' 30.5"
Longitude W 108° 59' 1.4"

THERE'S ONE REALLY GOOD THING about staying at Fulford Cave Campground: if it rains, you aren't necessarily tent bound. You can take advantage of rainy time as a chance to explore Fulford Cave itself, which is less than a mile from this intimate campground. Fulford Cave Campground is in an unusual setting and has other trails leading into the western side of the Holy Cross Wilderness, one of Colorado's best wild places.

The hilltop campground is on the left flank of the East Brush Creek Valley, in a scattered forest of aspen, spruce, and fir. Directly up the watershed is Craig Peak. Below you is the meadow of Yeoman Park. Off to your right, a few hundred feet down a steep rockslide, is East Brush Creek. Just behind the campground is a beaver pond. Off to your left are the trailhead to Fulford Cave and the other trails leading into the Holy Cross Wilderness.

As the forest road dead ends, the campground is straight ahead and the Fulford Cave trailhead parking is off to your left. A small spur road splits to the right, where the first three campsites lie. The first one is right on the edge of the drop into East Brush Creek. Be careful after dark if you camp here. The other two sites are by themselves and out of view over a little knob; they offer the most in campsite privacy.

The other four campsites are on a little loop road just as you pull up. One site is in the center of the loop, along with the vault toilet. Two water spigots are available at this diminutive campground. No self-respecting RV or pop-up camper would try to fit in these tent-only campsites. The bigger rigs stay just down the road at Yeoman Park Campground, where you should camp if Fulford Cave ever fills (which it rarely does).

Fulford Cave is Colorado's eighth-largest cavern. More than 2,600 square feet of the underground location

> *Fulford Cave offers attractions both above and below ground. The camping is above ground.*

RATINGS

Beauty: ✪ ✪ ✪
Privacy: ✪ ✪ ✪
Spaciousness: ✪ ✪
Quiet: ✪ ✪ ✪ ✪
Security: ✪ ✪ ✪
Cleanliness: ✪ ✪ ✪

ADDRESS: Fulford Cave
Campground
Eagle Ranger
District
P.O. Box 720
125 West Fifth Street
Eagle, CO 81631

OPERATED BY: USDA Forest
Service, White River
National Forest

INFORMATION: (970) 328-6388;
www.fs.fed.us/r2/
whiteriver

OPEN: June–October

SITES: 7

EACH SITE HAS: Picnic table, fire pit

ASSIGNMENT: First come,
first served; no
reservation

REGISTRATION: Self-registration on
site

FACILITIES: Water spigot, vault
toilet, summer trash
collection

PARKING: At campsites only

FEE: $8 per night

ELEVATION: 9,400 feet

RESTRICTIONS: *Pets:* On leash only
Fires: In fire pits only
Alcohol: At campsites
only
Vehicles: 25 feet
Other: 14-day stay
limit

has been plotted. Inside are big rooms, narrow crevices, streams, stalagmites, and stalactites. (Harken back to your school days and try to remember which one develops from the top down and which one builds from the bottom up.) Fulford Cave was discovered during the mining boom of the nineteenth century by a man named Maxwell, who named the cave after the nearby mining town of Fulford. He never found the riches he sought in the cave, but he did leave a timbered entrance and a pit entrance.

The 0.7-mile trail to the cave starts by the gate at the trailhead parking area. Start making your way up the forest on switchbacks, and you'll soon come to the cave. If you do explore inside the cave, the Forest Service recommends you have the following with you: durable and warm clothing, gloves, hard hat, flashlights and head lamps, sturdy boots, and drinking water. A cave map is available at the Ranger Station in Eagle. Remember, just like on the surface, you are responsible for your own safety in the cave.

Speaking of on the surface, there are two good trails that head into the Holy Cross Wilderness from Fulford Cave. They both lead to 16-acre Lake Charles. The Lake Charles Trail follows East Brush Creek for 4.4 miles before coming to the lake. Mystic Island Lake is a mile farther. Both lakes offer good fishing for cutthroat trout, while East Brush Creek offers fishing for rainbow, brook, and brown trout. I recommend fishing the stream in the meadows and beaver ponds below Fulford Cave.

The Ironedge Trail is a horse and foot trail. It offers many highlights on its 7-mile journey, as the surroundings change from aspen to fir to alpine tundra above the tree line. Along the way are cabins, meadows, and mine sites, interspersed with good views. The last two miles are downhill to Lake Charles. You can combine the Ironedge Trail with the Lake Charles Trail to make an excellent loop hike. For this particular adventure, you don't need a hardhat.

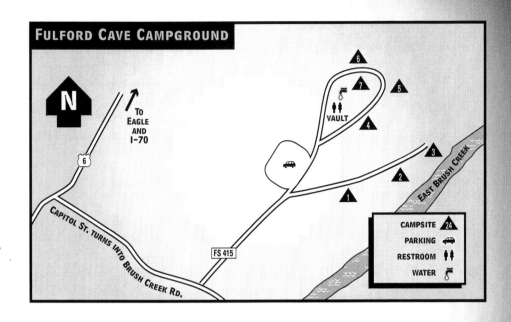

FULFORD CAVE CAMPGROUND

CAMPSITE 24
PARKING
RESTROOM
WATER

GETTING THERE

From the I-70 exit in Eagle, head south on US 6 as it veers right and then make a sharp left on Capitol Street. Proceed on Capitol Street as it turns into Brush Creek Road for 10 miles and come to FS 415 (East Brush Creek Road). Turn left on FS 415 and follow it 7 miles to Fulford Cave Campground.

GPS COORDINATES

UTM Zone (WGS84)	13S
Easting	0357450
Northing	4372620
Latitude	N 39° 29' 29.5"
Longitude	W 106° 39' 28.0"

THE BEST
IN TENT
CAMPING
COLORADO

> *If you really want to get away from it all, come here. You'll see a whole different side of Colorado.*

IRISH **CANYON IS FOR ADVENTUROUS** tent campers. It is off the beaten path and then some, in the extreme northwest corner of the state on Bureau of Land Management (BLM) land. This is in the Browns Park area, where Butch Cassidy and his gang retreated to safety between heists at the turn of the century. Irish Canyon itself is named for a trio of robbers who lit down the gorge after a hold-up in nearby Rock Springs, Wyoming.

These days you can enjoy the scenery and solitude of Irish Canyon, then venture out to a host of sights including Indian petroglyphs, Vermillion Falls, Lodore Hall, Browns Park National Wildlife Refuge, the Gates of Lodore, and more.

Irish Canyon is only 100 yards wide as you enter it. High rock walls drop down to sage, grass, and boulder fields. Gnarled old piñon and juniper trees rise along the wall in places. When you come to the campground, the sage gives way to old trees that climb up Cold Spring Mountain. Across the canyon is a sharp, high wall of rock, where small trees cling to precipices. I arrived at Irish Canyon in the afternoon, when the sun burned so brightly into the wall it shone. Later, a full moon rose over the canyon, making it easy to imagine outlaws tending stolen cattle rustled into the gorge.

A teardrop loop enters the forest of old juniper and piñon, above a campsite that overlooks the quiet road traversing the canyon. This site has two tables for larger groups. The second site also overlooks the flat below and the immense wall, but has ample shade.

The campsites farther up the loop are more secluded. The campsite atop the loop is large and is the most private. Three more campsites occupy somewhat leveled areas on the way back down. The picnic table pads have all been leveled, but some tent sites have a slight slope to them. A single vault toilet lies in

RATINGS

Beauty: ✿ ✿ ✿ ✿ ✿
Privacy: ✿ ✿ ✿
Spaciousness: ✿ ✿ ✿
Quiet: ✿ ✿ ✿ ✿
Security: ✿ ✿
Cleanliness: ✿ ✿ ✿

the wooded interior of the loop for all to use. No water is provided; you must bring your own. Browns Store, 10 miles from the camp and west down CO 318, has water, gas, a phone, and limited supplies. They also rent out canoes if you want to float down a quiet section of the Green River.

This is a very isolated camp; but with a road alongside it. So if you worry about leaving your gear unattended, have your adventures, then set up camp and stay there. This area no longer hosts robbers; most passers-by are friendly local ranchers, so you needn't be concerned about theft. Nor should you be concerned with Irish Canyon filling up. Campsites are available year-round.

At a place like Irish Canyon, you have to explore and make your own adventures. There are no rangers to tell you what to do or brochures laying everything out. It is wise to contact the BLM office in Craig for information to help you plan exactly what you want to do.

On your way from Maybell, watch for signs leading to local sights and make note of their particular roads. The old coke ovens are near Greystone. The Sand Wash Basin has a herd of wild horses. On the way in, stop at Vermillion Falls. It's a pretty, yet strange, sight—a cascade in such dry land. On old jeep roads, you can also explore by foot or mountain bike Vermillion Creek and its colorful, badlands canyon. The Gates of Lodore is the entrance to a magnificent canyon, where the Green River leaves Browns Park and crashes downstream to meet the Yampa River at Dinosaur National Monument. A trail leaves the picnic area at the entrance of the canyon to see some Indian petroglyphs, possibly inscribed by two different tribes on the same rock.

The hiking and mountain biking around Irish Canyon is limited only by your stamina. Marked trails are few, but jeep roads are many. Below the canyon, paths lead up Green Canyon onto Peek-a-boo Ridge and a sweeping view of Browns Park below. Old jeep roads lead up Talamantes Creek farther up the canyon onto Cold Spring Mountain. Unless on foot, stay on the roads.

KEY INFORMATION

ADDRESS: Irish Canyon Campground Little Snake BLM Field Office 455 Emerson Street Craig, CO 81625

OPERATED BY: Bureau of Land Management

INFORMATION: (970) 826-5087 or (970) 826-5000; www.co.blm.gov/lsra/camping.htm

OPEN: All year

SITES: 6

EACH SITE HAS: Picnic table, steel fire ring

ASSIGNMENT: First come, first served; no reservation

REGISTRATION: No registration

FACILITIES: Vault toilet (bring water)

PARKING: At campsites only

FEE: No fee

ELEVATION: 6,650 feet

RESTRICTIONS: *Pets:* On leash only
Fires: In fire rings only
Alcohol: At campsites only
Vehicles: 30 feet, on roads only
Other: 14-day stay limit

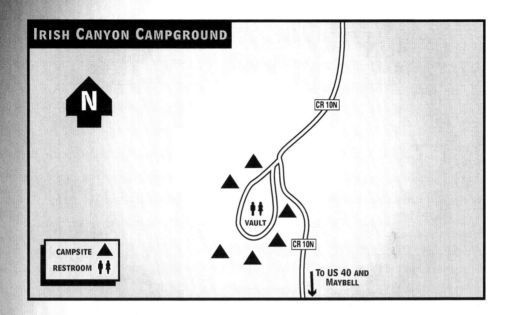

IRISH CANYON CAMPGROUND

N

CR 10N

VAULT

CR 10N

CAMPSITE

RESTROOM

To US 40 AND
MAYBELL

GETTING THERE

From Maybell, drive west on US 40 for 0.5 mile, then turn right on CO 318 and follow it for 41 miles to CR 10N. Turn right on CR 10N and follow it 8 miles to Irish Canyon Campground, which will be on your left.

Drive down to Browns Park National Wildlife Refuge to absorb a little human and natural history. Thousands of birds stop here during spring and fall migration. Elk and deer make this ribbon of green their home during the winter. You can make the 11-mile auto tour of the refuge and see the old Lodore Hall, where you'll find another petroglyph rock and the Two Bar Ranch. This was the stomping ground of Butch Cassidy. Thanks to the proximity of three states, Colorado, Utah, and Wyoming, ruffians could slip across state lines and out of jurisdiction when lawmen chased them.

I loved this area; finding it was a steal, better than the loot Butch Cassidy and the Wild Bunch were after.

GPS COORDINATES

UTM Zone (WGS84)   12T
Easting   0690930
Northing   4522220
Latitude   N 40° 49' 44.1"
Longitude   W 108° 44' 8.5"

TRY THIS ONE ON FOR SIZE: Colorado's favorite year-round waterfall was created from limestone buildup behind an ancient beaver dam, and these are the cliffs we see today. The falls became a 19th-century tourist attraction and was then used as the impetus for Colorado's first hydroelectric plant. The plant was then dismantled and a state park was built around the picturesque site. The state later renovated the park and campground into what we see today. Bet you didn't know beavers could be that constructive.

No matter how the falls came to be—and I am skeptical about that beaver dam story—the falls are here now and you can delight in them and the lakes of Rifle Gap State Park, Harvey Gap State Park, rock climbing at Rifle Mountain Park, the East Fork Rifle State Fish Hatchery, and more outdoor recreation in the White River National Forest nearby. All this can be enjoyed from your base camp at the pleasing walk-in tent sites set in the riparian lushness of the East Fork Rifle Creek.

Park your car at Rifle Falls and take the Squirrel Trail that runs along East Fork Rifle Creek. The campsites spur off the Squirrel Trail. The first campsite is set beneath tall, narrow leaf cottonwoods and is the only site not along the creek. Continue on and you'll find more sites scattered among the box elder, willow, grass, and cottonwoods of the creek bottom.

All the sites have been renovated and are more appealing than ever. Each campsite is completely separated from the rest; the farther down the path, the more separated the sites become. The stream sends out a constant symphony of whitewater music. The final campsite is mostly surrounded by the creek, and it is the most isolated and one of the best tent sites in the entire state park system.

> *Rifle Falls is the scenic centerpiece of the Rifle Valley. Set up your base camp here and explore the nearby parks and forest land.*

RATINGS

Beauty: ✿ ✿ ✿ ✿
Privacy: ✿ ✿ ✿ ✿ ✿
Spaciousness: ✿ ✿ ✿ ✿
Quiet: ✿ ✿ ✿
Security: ✿ ✿ ✿ ✿ ✿
Cleanliness: ✿ ✿ ✿ ✿

ADDRESS: Rifle Falls State Park
Campground
00050 Road 219
Rifle, CO 81650

OPERATED BY: Colorado State Parks

INFORMATION: (970) 625-1607;
parks.state.co.us;
rifle.gap.park
@state.co.us

OPEN: All year

SITES: 7 walk-in tent sites
(Squirrel), 13 drive-
in sites (Falls)

EACH SITE HAS: Walk-in sites have
picnic table, fire
grate, tent pad;
drive-in sites have
picnic table, fire
grate, electricity

ASSIGNMENT: By reservation or
pick an available
site on arrival

REGISTRATION: (800) 678-CAMP (2267)
or (303) 470-1144
in metro Denver,
at park entrance,
or www.reserve
america.com

FACILITIES: Water spigot, vault
toilets

PARKING: At campsites only

FEE: $5 Parks Pass plus
$12 per night tent
sites, $16 per night
drive-in sites; an
additional $8 fee
added to each
reservation

ELEVATION: 6,500 feet

RESTRICTIONS: *Pets:* On leash only
Fires: In fire grates
only
Alcohol: 3.2% beer
only
Vehicles: None
Other: 14-day stay
limit

Thirteen drive-in sites comprise the balance of the campground, which caters to RVs. These sites have been renovated as well and the whole campground has a tidy appearance to it that meets the high standards of Colorado state parks. Water spigots and new vault toilets have been built to serve the area.

If you want to stay here, get a reservation. There is no reason not to make the five-minute phone call to eliminate the horror of a full campground. Get a reservation no matter when you come. This campground is open year-round.

Of course, Rifle Falls will probably be your first visit. Feel the mist as water plunges down three chutes to the pool below. Take the trail to the top of the falls and see the caves that are there too. Another hiking opportunity is the Squirrel Trail, which crosses the creek below the falls and explores the waterside lushness of this valley.

Speaking of water, if you vie for trout in the creek and none bite, head a short ways up the valley to the state fish hatchery. They are open for visitation and at least you can take a look at a trout—actually hundreds of them.

Farther up the valley is Rifle Mountain Park. This is where the rock climbers do their work, scaling the sheer walls of the East Fork Rifle Creek canyon. Even if climbing isn't your thing, check out the free show and admire their bravado. Anglers take note that the creek is stocked up here. Farther up the creek is the White River National Forest. The Three Forks Trail leaves Three Forks Campground and makes a loop up by Coulter Lake back to the Spruce Picnic Area.

Below Rifle Falls is Rifle Gap State Park. Boaters and jet skiers make wakes through the 350-acre impoundment, and there is a swimming beach for those who like their water sports a little slower. The fishing here can be fast or slow, depending on your skill and luck, of course. Harvey Gap State Park offers more aquatic pleasures and is just a few miles away. There is no waterskiing here; you are more likely to see windsurfers cutting a wake. The 160-acre lake has trout and warm-water fish such as smallmouth bass and crappie.

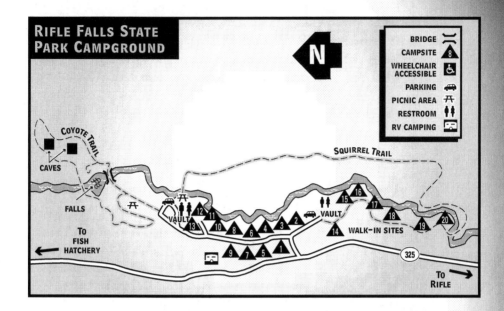

RIFLE FALLS STATE PARK CAMPGROUND

Map legend:
- BRIDGE
- CAMPSITE
- WHEELCHAIR ACCESSIBLE
- PARKING
- PICNIC AREA
- RESTROOM
- RV CAMPING

COYOTE TRAIL
CAVES
SQUIRREL TRAIL
FALLS
VAULT
WALK-IN SITES
To FISH HATCHERY
325
To RIFLE

The city of Rifle is nearby for any supplies you might need, so pitch your tent at the falls and enjoy all there is to enjoy in this little Colorado valley with a big punch.

GETTING THERE

From Rifle, go north on CO 13 for 3 miles. Turn right onto CO 325 and drive 9.8 miles.

GPS COORDINATES

UTM Zone (WGS84)	13S
Easting	0268190
Northing	4393820
Latitude	N 39° 39' 46.0"
Longitude	W 107° 42' 8.7"

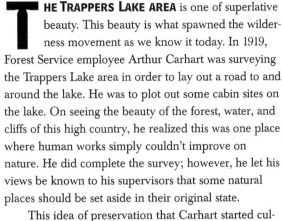

> *This is the best tent campground at Trappers Lake, birthplace of the wilderness movement.*

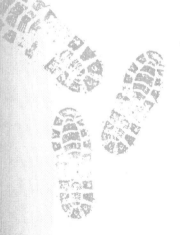

THE **TRAPPERS LAKE AREA** is one of superlative beauty. This beauty is what spawned the wilderness movement as we know it today. In 1919, Forest Service employee Arthur Carhart was surveying the Trappers Lake area in order to lay out a road to and around the lake. He was to plot out some cabin sites on the lake. On seeing the beauty of the forest, water, and cliffs of this high country, he realized this was one place where human works simply couldn't improve on nature. He did complete the survey; however, he let his views be known to his supervisors that some natural places should be set aside in their original state.

This idea of preservation that Carhart started culminated in the Wilderness Act of 1964; today there are more than 3 million acres of wilderness land set aside in Colorado alone. The nearest wilderness, the Flat Tops Wilderness, nearly encircles Trappers Lake. There are several campgrounds in the immediate Trappers Lake area, but Shepherds Rim is the best campground for tent campers.

Shepherds Rim is set in a thick spruce forest that is left intact wherever possible, integrating the campground into the woods. A slight slope has required the Forest Service to erect retaining walls and some steps between the road and the actual camping areas to level the campsites, making them more camper-friendly.

With several small campsites and parking spots, the layout of Shepherds Rim discourages the bigger rigs from camping here, despite the presence of a few drive-through campsites. In general, the abundance of tent pads means a majority of overnight visitors are tent campers.

Enter the long and narrow campground loop, then pass the first drive-through camp-site (even though it is drive-through, it also has a tent pad). Most of the campsites are on the outside of the loop, increasing privacy.

RATINGS

Beauty: ✿ ✿ ✿ ✿
Privacy: ✿ ✿ ✿
Spaciousness: ✿ ✿ ✿
Quiet: ✿ ✿ ✿
Security: ✿ ✿ ✿ ✿ ✿
Cleanliness: ✿ ✿ ✿ ✿

Short paths connect parking areas to the picnic tables to the tent pads. The tent pads are often farther back in the woods, making for better privacy.

The sites at the back of the loop are the most private. There is a special handicapped-accessible site, a double campsite for larger parties, and a campground host to make your stay safe and pleasant. Overall, the Forest Service has upgraded this spot into a well-kept, quality campground that you can use as a base camp to enjoy this area.

Water recreation centers around Trappers Lake, more than 300 acres of picturesque Flat Tops splendor. Cliffs rise above the forest and reflect off the clear, clean tarn, where brook and native cutthroat trout thrive. No motors are allowed here, so bring a paddle along with your canoe to enjoy the peaceful environment. Fishing is by artificial flies and lures only. Possession limit is eight for the nearly pure strain of cutthroats. There is no possession limit on brook trout. Other fishing opportunities are along the North Fork of the White River below Trappers Lake and along Fraser Creek, which feeds Trappers Lake.

You can combine hiking and fishing by using many of the trails that radiate from Trappers Lake into the surrounding Flat Tops Wilderness. The nearest trail to Shepherds Rim is the Wall Lake Trail, #1818. It leads up and away steeply from the campgrounds to reach the Flat Tops Plateau after 3 miles. Meadows and forest intermingle here. Wall Lake, 2 miles farther, offers fishing for cutthroat trout.

The Carhart Trail, #1815, roughly circles Trappers Lake in a 4.5-mile loop. It parallels the east and north shore of the lake, allowing for angling opportunities, but pulls away from the lake as it crosses Fraser Creek to intersect the Wall Lake Trail. The Stillwater Lake Trail spurs off the Carhart Trail and heads east to Little Trappers Lake and other fishable lakes. It also offers views of the Chinese Wall, an impressive blockade of rock that extends for miles.

Buy all your supplies before coming to Trappers Lake, then plan to stay a while. This body of water and the surrounding Flat Tops are among the best locations in the state—and that is saying a lot.

KEY INFORMATION

ADDRESS:	Shepherds Rim Campground Blanco Ranger District 317 East Market Street Meeker, CO 81641
OPERATED BY:	USDA Forest Service, White River National Forest
INFORMATION:	(970) 878-4039; www.fs.fed.us/r2/ whiteriver
OPEN:	June or July– September
SITES:	17
EACH SITE HAS:	Picnic table, fire grate, some tent pads
ASSIGNMENT:	First come, first served; no reservation
REGISTRATION:	Self-registration on-site
FACILITIES:	Water spigot, vault toilet
PARKING:	At campsites only
FEE:	$15 per night
ELEVATION:	9,900 feet
RESTRICTIONS:	*Pets:* On leash only *Fires:* In fire grates only *Alcohol:* At campsites only *Vehicles:* 36 feet *Other:* 10-day stay limit; campground borders the wilderness; please obey all wilderness regulations

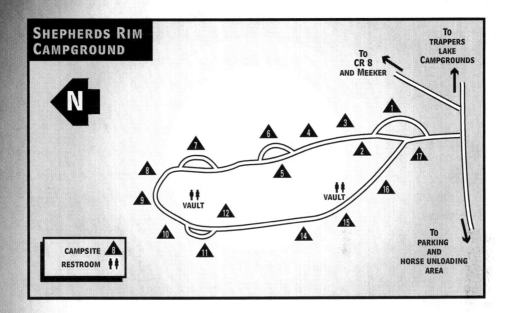

GETTING THERE

From Meeker, travel east 1 mile on CO 13. Turn right onto CR 8 to Trappers Lake Road. Travel 11 miles to the campgrounds. Turn right. Shepherds Rim will be 1 mile on the right.

GPS COORDINATES

UTM Zone (WGS84)   13S
Easting   0308650
Northing   4429480
Latitude   N 39° 59' 37.5"
Longitude   W 107° 14' 29"

SOME PLACES GET REPUTATIONS. As I scoured the state in search of the best tent campgrounds, Steamboat Lake kept coming up as an unquestionable inclusion for this book. I was expecting something special, and I wasn't disappointed. It started with the new Visitor Center and ended with the view from the walk-in tent sites from Bridge Island. In between was the town of Steamboat Springs—in my opinion Colorado's most attractive resort—Hahn's Peak, Pearl Lake, and the Mount Zirkel Wilderness.

Don't be turned off by the large number of campsites here. They are divided over two major campgrounds. The tent area is set apart on an island and is the main concern to us tent campers.

The Sunrise Vista Campground has 113 sites on the eastern edge of Steamboat Lake. If you are going to stay here, try the Harebell Loop. There will be big rigs here, but this loop nevertheless offers the closest lakeside campsites at Sunrise Vista. The Larkspur Loop is well shaded. The Yarrow Loop also has some lakeside sites, but is dominated by RVs.

The Dutch Hill Campground has 85 campsites. The Wheeler and Baker Loops have electric hookups and are dominated by RVs. Pass the camper services building (with showers, laundry, and so on) near the marina, then arrive at Bridge Island, tent camper's heaven. The first 15 campsites are on a loop beneath lodgepole pines. These are drive-up sites that are a little too crowded for my taste. But they are on the island, and the eight campsites on the outside of the loop are near the water.

But the best is last: On the far side of this loop is the parking area for the tent-only campsites. These last 20 sites occupy the part of the island that juts out far-thest into Steamboat Lake. The walk to the campsites ranges anywhere from 20 to 200 feet, but the lake and

> *You can enjoy not only all that this state park offers but also thousands of acres of surrounding national forest and the resort town of Steamboat Springs.*

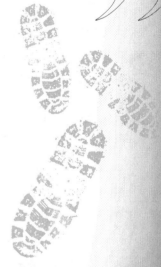

RATINGS

Beauty: ✩ ✩ ✩ ✩
Privacy: ✩ ✩ ✩
Spaciousness: ✩ ✩ ✩ ✩
Quiet: ✩ ✩ ✩
Security: ✩ ✩ ✩ ✩ ✩
Cleanliness: ✩ ✩ ✩ ✩

ADDRESS: Steamboat Lake
State Park
Campground
Box 750
Clark, CO 80428

OPERATED BY: Colorado State Parks

INFORMATION: (970) 879-3922;
parks.state.co.us/
steamboat; steam
boat@state.co.us

OPEN: Mid-May–October

SITES: 20 walk-in tent only,
198 others

EACH SITE HAS: Picnic table, fire
grate, tent pad;
55 others have
electricity also

ASSIGNMENT: By reservation or
pick an available
site on arrival

REGISTRATION: (800) 678-CAMP (2267)
or (303) 470-1144
in metro Denver,
at www.reserve
america.com, or at
campground booth

FACILITIES: Hot showers, flush
and vault toilets,
laundry, phone,
vending machines,
marina store

PARKING: At campsites or
walk-in tent campers
parking area

FEE: $5 Parks Pass plus
$12–$14 per night
walk-in tent sites or
nonelectric vehicle
sites, $16–$18 per
night electric vehicle
sites

ELEVATION: 8,100 feet

RESTRICTIONS: *Pets:* On leash only
Fires: In fire grates
Alcohol: 3.2% beer
only
Other: 14-day stay
limit

mountain views get better the farther you are from the parking area.

The walk-in campsites are situated in wooded areas between fields that are far from one another. A gravel path spurs off the main gravel loop, connecting the campsites. The sites are dispersed so that campers on the interior of the loop have a quality view as well. The southernmost campsites are the best and most isolated. Boaters can actually pull their craft onto the shore of the island and walk to their campsites.

As the loop swings around, the campsites enter heavy lodgepole woods. The view is across to the marina. These are the least desirable, but still good, walk-in sites. Two vault toilets serve the immediate area, though full facilities are nearby at the camper service building.

If you want to stay here, get a reservation, though the tent sites are the last to be filled. This park has a strong following among the locals, which speaks volumes about its quality. Front Range campers make the drive to overnight here, so do out-of-staters. I repeat, make a reservation to secure a campsite.

Steamboat Lake is, naturally, a park attraction. All manner of water sports are enjoyed on the lake. Skiers, anglers, and personal watercraft enthusiasts use the reservoir. A power zone and a no-wake zone make Steamboat Lake enjoyable for all park visitors. The inlets of the lake offer the best fishing for rainbow, brown, arctic grayling, and native cutthroat trout. If you didn't bring your own watercraft, anything from canoes to pontoon boats can be rented at the park marina, where they also have limited supplies.

Nearby Pearl Lake is another scenic component of the state park system. It offers trout fishing on a smaller reservoir. This is a wakeless lake, so it's a quieter fishing destination.

If you want to get around on foot, first hop in your car and enjoy the Routt National Forest, which nearly encircles Steamboat Lake. Hahn's Peak is a popular hike. The Mount Zirkel Wilderness is east of Steamboat Lake. The Slavonia trailhead is your best bet for enjoying this glacier-carved highland, where hundreds of alpine lakes dot the landscape. Take the Slavonia Trail

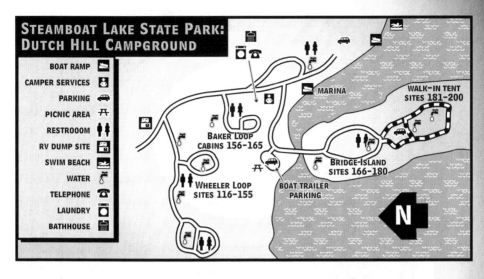

STEAMBOAT LAKE STATE PARK: DUTCH HILL CAMPGROUND

BOAT RAMP	
CAMPER SERVICES	
PARKING	
PICNIC AREA	
RESTROOOM	
RV DUMP SITE	
SWIM BEACH	
WATER	
TELEPHONE	
LAUNDRY	
BATHHOUSE	

MARINA

WALK-IN TENT
SITES 181-200

BAKER LOOP
CABINS 156-165

BRIDGE-ISLAND
SITES 166-180

WHEELER LOOP
SITES 116-155

BOAT TRAILER
PARKING

N

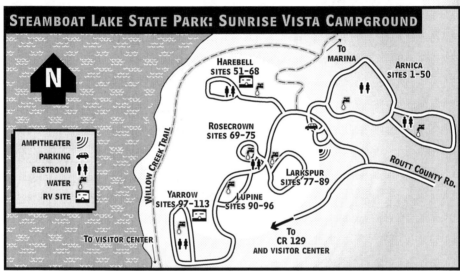

STEAMBOAT LAKE STATE PARK: SUNRISE VISTA CAMPGROUND

N

HAREBELL
SITES 51-68

TO
MARINA

ARNICA
SITES 1-50

ROSECROWN
SITES 69-75

AMPITHEATER	
PARKING	
RESTROOM	
WATER	
RV SITE	

WILLOW CREEK TRAIL

LARKSPUR
SITES 77-89

ROUTT COUNTY RD.

YARROW
SITES 97-113

LUPINE
SITES 90-96

TO VISITOR CENTER

TO
CR 129
AND VISITOR CENTER

up to Gilpin Lake, then loop back down Gold Creek. The Encampment River and North Fork Elk River offer hiking and angling opportunities. A map is sold in the Routt National Forest Visitor Center, which has over 2,000 square feet of interpretive displays.

GETTING THERE

From Steamboat Springs, drive west on US 40 for 2 miles to CR 129. Turn right on CR 129 and follow it north for 26 miles to Steamboat Lake State Park.

GPS COORDINATES

UTM Zone (WGS84) 13T

Easting 0333990

Northing 4519490

Latitude N 40° 48' 35.4"

Longitude W 106° 58' 5.3"

31
WEIR AND JOHNSON CAMPGROUND

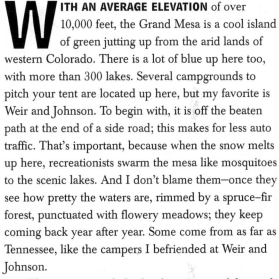

> *Lakes are plentiful, and the camping is fine here on top of the Grand Mesa.*

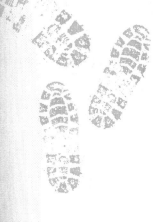

WITH AN AVERAGE ELEVATION of over 10,000 feet, the Grand Mesa is a cool island of green jutting up from the arid lands of western Colorado. There is a lot of blue up here too, with more than 300 lakes. Several campgrounds to pitch your tent are located up here, but my favorite is Weir and Johnson. To begin with, it is off the beaten path at the end of a side road; this makes for less auto traffic. That's important, because when the snow melts up here, recreationists swarm the mesa like mosquitoes to the scenic lakes. And I don't blame them—once they see how pretty the waters are, rimmed by a spruce–fir forest, punctuated with flowery meadows; they keep coming back year after year. Some come from as far as Tennessee, like the campers I befriended at Weir and Johnson.

This campground also lies between two lakes and has trails leaving the campground to access three more lakes. These lakes are in addition to countless other lakes and the Crag Crest National Scenic Trail that is accessible by auto.

If you have successfully driven to the campground without stopping to wet your fishing line, enter the campground loop. Off to your left are two campsites that are in an area where the Engelmann spruce and subalpine fir have been thinned a bit. As you continue the loop, the western tip of Weir and Johnson Reservoir is off to your right. A third campsite sits across the road from the lake.

As the loop curves, a small cascade rushes downhill past four excellent tent sites down from the loop road beside Sackett Reservoir. You have to carry your gear a bit to reach them, but you are that much closer to the aquamarine water. The next two sites are also down near Sackett Reservoir. The final three campsites are away from the lake, but are heavily shaded.

RATINGS

Beauty: ✪ ✪ ✪
Privacy: ✪ ✪ ✪
Spaciousness: ✪ ✪ ✪
Quiet: ✪ ✪ ✪ ✪
Security: ✪ ✪ ✪
Cleanliness: ✪ ✪ ✪

On my early July visit, one campsite was still too snow-covered to use!

There is a pair of vault toilets for campers. The old pump well is capped—bring your own water and you won't have to take any chances.

You will be taking chances if you try to camp here on July 4 or Labor Day. Weekends can fill, but if you get here by mid–Friday afternoon, you should get a campsite. Campsites are nearly always available during the week.

Trout swim the waters of the two campground reservoirs, and fishing is popular throughout the Grand Mesa, but hike-in lakes often see less fishing pressure. You can walk to Leon Lake. Just cross the Weir and Johnson Dam, hug the shoreline to the right, and cross a small pass to Leon Lake, which is larger than Weir and Johnson. Round Lake and Leon Peak Reservoir are nearby too. Cross the Weir and Johnson Reservoir dam, then bear left when the trail splits.

After seeing all these lakes, I was wishing for my canoe. Bring yours, or borrow one; you can really get around to less-fished spots on all these lakes up here, nearly 2 miles high. And there is hardly more scenic paddling in the state. If you bring a motorboat, check the regulations—many lakes are too small for motorized craft and don't allow them.

Hiking "The Crag" is tops for foot travel on the Grand Mesa. The Crag Crest National Scenic Trail is a 6.5-mile path that rides the spine of the mesa and offers views in all directions of far-off mountain ranges. On this inspiring hike, you can see all the lakes lying below you like emerald jewels in the forest. The Crag Crest Connector Trail passes through forest and meadow to complete a 10-mile circuit. You can pick up "the Crag" back on FS 121 near The Crag Crest Campground, which you passed on the way in.

More information can be obtained at the Grand Mesa Visitor Center at the junction of Colorado 65 and FS 121. Supplies can be purchased at a small store a couple of miles east on FS 121 from the Visitor Center.

KEY INFORMATION

ADDRESS:	Weir and Johnson Campground Grand Valley Ranger District 277 Crossroads Boulevard, Suite A Grand Junction, CO 81506
OPERATED BY:	USDA Forest Service, Grand Mesa, Uncompahgre, and Gunnison National Forests
INFORMATION:	(970) 242-8211; www.fs.fed.us/r2/gmug
OPEN:	July–late September
SITES:	12
EACH SITE HAS:	Picnic table, fire grate
ASSIGNMENT:	First come, first served; no reservation
REGISTRATION:	No registration
FACILITIES:	Vault toilets
PARKING:	At campsites only
FEE:	None
ELEVATION:	10,500 feet
RESTRICTIONS:	*Pets:* On leash only *Fires:* In fire grates only *Alcohol:* Allowed *Vehicles:* 20 feet *Other:* 14-day stay limit

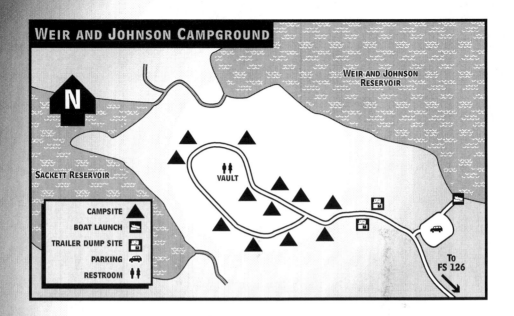

GETTING THERE

From Cedaredge, head north on CO 65 for 15 miles to FS 121. Turn right on FS 121 and follow it for 9 miles to FS 126. Turn right on FS 126 and follow it 3 miles to the dead end at Weir and Johnson Campground.

GPS COORDINATES

UTM Zone (WGS84)   13S
Easting   0255034
Northing   4328017
Latitude   N 39° 4' 0.9"
Longitude   W 107° 49' 53.0"

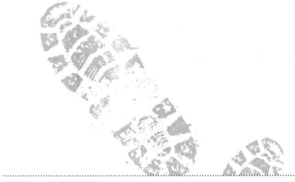

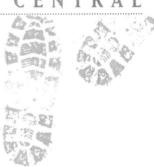

SOUTH CENTRAL **COLORADO**

32
ALVARADO CAMPGROUND

ALVARADO IS AN ACTIVE PERSON'S campground. On a summer Saturday there will be hikers, bikers, and horseback riders gearing up and heading out on their favorite trails. Several of the trails leave directly from the campground, which is a nice place to return after a day in the scenic Sangre de Cristo Mountains.

Alvarado meets the banner standard set by the Sangre de Cristos. On a slope just into the forest line above the Wet Mountain Valley, Alvarado enjoys a mixture of woodland and meadow, where Douglas fir and ponderosa pines intermingle with aspen. Cottonwood and brush grow thick along Alvarado Creek. Forest density varies with exposure on the three loops. So no matter what your preference for sun or shade, view or privacy, your wishes should be fulfilled, unless it is a weekend holiday, the only time the campground fills.

The first few campsites are in a meadow overlooking the mountains across the valley, then the main road enters a ponderosa grove. The right-hand road, with several nice campsites along it, leads to the Venable trailhead, which is located at the end of this loop. The main campground road continues upward, with campsites on a rocky slope beneath the pines. Another road splits off to the right into a grove of aspen. It has several campsites that offer much shade and some views of Comanche Mountain, high in the Sangre de Cristos above. The road switchbacks farther up the mountain with more shaded and isolated campsites, then comes to a set of five walk-in, tent-only sites. Here, you park your car and walk a short distance to set up camp. But these sites are on a slope and you may be hard-pressed to find a level place to pitch your tent. However, the entire campground is suitable for tents. This road ends at a turnaround and the Comanche trailhead.

> *Alvarado is on the eastern slope of the Sangre de Cristo Mountains.*

RATINGS

Beauty: ✿ ✿ ✿ ✿
Privacy: ✿ ✿ ✿ ✿
Spaciousness: ✿ ✿ ✿
Quiet: ✿ ✿ ✿
Security: ✿ ✿ ✿ ✿
Cleanliness: ✿ ✿ ✿ ✿

KEY INFORMATION

The final set of campsites are on a side road of their own in a ponderosa grove off the main campground road. Water spigots and vault toilets are spread throughout the campground, which is very large to have only 47 campsites. Many of the sites are spread quite far apart. A campground host is stationed at the entrance to the campground for your safety.

Hikers, bikers, and horse riders all enjoy the area trails, most of which lead into the far-flung Sangre de Cristo Wilderness. The Comanche Trail heads up along Alvarado Creek to Comanche Lake. The Venable Trail leads up a couple of miles to Venable Falls, then a few more miles to the Venable Lakes areas. Most of these lakes don't thaw out until late June. You can combine the Comanche and Venable trails and make a strenuous 13-mile loop via Phantom Terrace back to the campground.

If you are looking to stretch your legs but not climb straight uphill, try the Rainbow Trail. It runs 46 miles all the way from south of Alvarado north to Salida. You can use the Rainbow Trail to connect to other trails entering the Sangre de Cristo Wilderness. The Godwin Trail, one watershed north, climbs to alpine lakes. The Cottonwood Trail, one watershed south, climbs along Cottonwood Creek. Any of these bodies of water are suitable for fishing.

You can also drive to within a quarter mile of Hermit Lake, another alpine body of water high in the mountains. Take County Road 160 (Hermit Road) west out of Westcliffe and drive 13 miles to a signed parking area near the lake. Bring your fishing pole.

You can reward yourself after all that exercise with a good meal at the Alpine Lodge, which is located a few steps from the campground. Or you can drive into Westcliffe and take the walking tour of the downtown area. Get your self-guiding brochure at the Tourist Information Center caboose. There is ample food, drink, and supplies here in town.

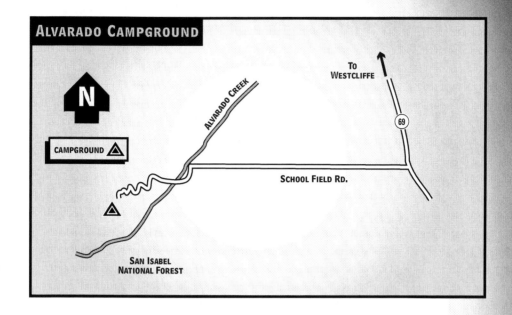

N

CAMPGROUND ▲

ALVARADO CREEK

TO
WESTCLIFFE

69

SCHOOL FIELD RD.

▲

SAN ISABEL
NATIONAL FOREST

GETTING THERE

From the courthouse in
Westcliffe, drive south on
CO 69 for 3 miles to CR 140
(School Field Road). Turn
right on CR 140 and follow
it for 6 miles to Alvarado
Campground.

GPS COORDINATES

UTM Zone (WGS84)   13S
Easting   0450180
Northing   4214766
Latitude   N 38° 4' 45.7"
Longitude   W 105° 34' 4.9"

33
BEAR LAKE CAMPGROUND

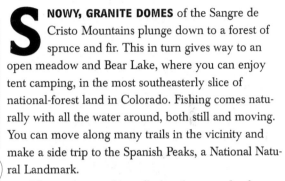

> *The magnificent Sangre de Cristo Mountains provide a scenic backdrop for Bear Lake.*

SNOWY, GRANITE DOMES of the Sangre de Cristo Mountains plunge down to a forest of spruce and fir. This in turn gives way to an open meadow and Bear Lake, where you can enjoy tent camping, in the most southeasterly slice of national-forest land in Colorado. Fishing comes naturally with all the water around, both still and moving. You can move along many trails in the vicinity and make a side trip to the Spanish Peaks, a National Natural Landmark.

The campground is well placed next to the dense forest and mountain meadow above Bear Lake. Along the campground's gravel loop, several wooded campsites are situated to your right with obscured views of Bear Lake. More open sites with occasional stray aspen are in the center of the loop as the road swings around into the grassy meadow. What these campsites lack in privacy they make up in views of Steep Mountain above, the nearby meadow, and a cathedral of peaks beyond. A few campsites on the outside of the loop face into the clearing, which has a stream flowing through it.

The Indian Creek trailhead starts just beyond campsite 9. The loop road begins to climb into the forest again. Another creek rushes from the high country through the campground to Bear Lake. The next few campsites are in the spur to your right, offering the most in campsite privacy.

This is one of the highest campgrounds around, so bring that extra blanket and expect to find temperatures around, or possibly below, freezing throughout the summer. Be prepared for windy, cool conditions any time at Bear Lake. Stake your tent down extra-taut as well, because the gusts of wind from the peaks above can blow mighty strong. Cover yourself from the penetrating rays of the sun. Experience taught me these lessons the hard way. On my visit I failed to

RATINGS

Beauty: ✿ ✿ ✿ ✿
Privacy: ✿ ✿
Spaciousness: ✿ ✿ ✿
Quiet: ✿ ✿ ✿ ✿
Security: ✿ ✿ ✿ ✿
Cleanliness: ✿ ✿ ✿ ✿

bring enough clothes for the chill, my face got sunburned, my tent was blown over, and I froze my tail off that night. And I still like this place.

Vault toilets are located at the center of the loop and near the Indian Creek trailhead. An old-fashioned pump provides water at the height of the campground. For your safety and security a campground host is situated at the beginning of the loop. Bring your supplies, as it is a far piece to the nearest full-service grocery store.

After setting up camp, why not check out Bear Lake? A foot trail circles the deep blue trout-laden water fed by streams from above. Drop in a line or two. No luck? Try Blue Lake. It's a mile by foot or road to the almost equally scenic fishing waters. You'll pass a few other small lakes along the way if you walk. For anglers who prefer moving water try fishing Cuchara Creek. It winds along Forest Service Road 422, your route up to Bear Lake.

Hikers have two nearby options in addition to Bear and Blue Lakes. Take the Indian Creek Trail from the campground north to Bonnet Park or make a loop via Baker and Dodgeton Creeks. Ambitious hikers will want to take the 3.5-mile gut-buster up the old North Fork four-wheel-drive road to Trinchera Peak (13,517 feet). The view will get your heart pumping again. This trek starts near Blue Lake.

Take your camera just south of Bear Lake on Colorado 12 to Cuchara Pass. FS 46 leads from the pass to the Spanish Peaks. These two granite domes are an offshoot of the Sangre de Cristo Mountains and will deliver scenery overload if you head to and beyond 11,000-foot Cordova Pass.

The isolation and long drive with no population base nearby make this a quiet campground, though there may be some site competition on summer holidays. Just come better prepared than I was.

KEY INFORMATION

ADDRESS: Bear Lake Campground San Carlos Ranger District 3170 East Main Street Cañon City, CO 81212

OPERATED BY: USDA Forest Service, Pike and San Isabel National Forests, Cimarron and Comanche National Grasslands

INFORMATION: (719) 269-8500; www.fs.fed.us/r2/psicc/sanc

OPEN: Memorial Day–mid-October

SITES: 15

EACH SITE HAS: Picnic table, fire grate, trash pick-up

ASSIGNMENT: First come, first served; no reservation

REGISTRATION: Self-registration on site

FACILITIES: Pump well water, vault toilets

PARKING: At campsites only

FEE: $13 per night

ELEVATION: 10,500 feet

RESTRICTIONS: *Pets:* On leash only
Fires: In fire grates only
Alcohol: At campsites only
Vehicles: 40-feet
Other: 14-day stay limit

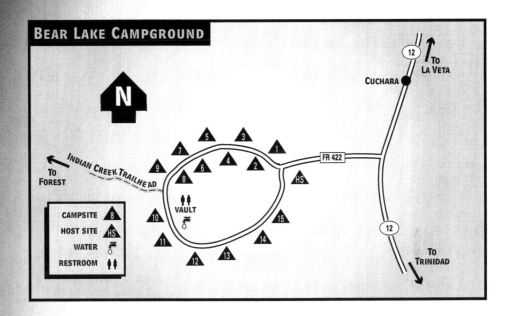

GETTING THERE

From La Veta, drive south
on CO 12 for 13 miles to
FS 422. Turn right on FS 422
and follow it for 5 miles to
Bear Lake Campground.

GPS COORDINATES

UTM Zone (WGS84)   13S
Easting   0487290
Northing   4131010
Latitude   N 37° 19' 32.5"
Longitude   W 105° 8' 36.0"

34
GREAT SAND DUNES NATIONAL PARK & PRESERVE: PINYON FLATS CAMPGROUND

I**T WAS AN INCREDIBLY WINDY DAY** as I headed toward the dunes. Dust and sand were blowing across the San Luis Valley. Blanca Peak towered on my right, somewhat clouded by the airborne grit. Later, the Great Sand Dunes appeared, a massive shifting swath of sand, contrasting with the verdant Sangre de Cristo Mountains in the background. The blustery day made it evident how such a peculiar sight could form in the middle of the Rocky Mountains.

Pinyon Flats Campground, located in the Great Sand Dunes National Park and Preserve, impressed me as well. It is set in a juniper–pine forest complemented with a sagebrush and grass understory between the dunes and the high country. There are two long, narrow loops, each with a variety of campsites to suit almost anyone. The Dunes Trail and seasonally flowing Garden Creek bisect the Pinyon Flats.

Loop A is lower and closer to the dunes. A paved road cuts down on dust. Low stone walls level the ground and define boundaries between the 44 campsites. Large rocks keep cars where they are supposed to be. Some campsites are nestled in piñon thickets, others are more open. But the open campsites offer views of the dunes and mountains. Most sites are spacious. As the loop circles back, campsites drop down from the road toward the dunes. These sunny sites offer incredible views of the sands, but they have a more worn and dusty appearance to them.

Loop B parallels Loop A, but is situated on higher, more wooded ground. It has 44 campsites as well and a few cottonwoods growing alongside Garden Creek, breaking up the evergreens. Elaborate rock work keeps the natural areas from being trampled and levels the campsites. Just beyond the Little Medano trailhead is a set of campsites that offers great views of the contrasting sand dunes and mountains.

> *You can't imagine the sight of America's largest sand dunes perched against the Rocky Mountains. Come see it for yourself.*

RATINGS

Beauty: ☆ ☆ ☆ ☆
Privacy: ☆ ☆ ☆
Spaciousness: ☆ ☆ ☆
Quiet: ☆ ☆ ☆
Security: ☆ ☆ ☆ ☆ ☆
Cleanliness: ☆ ☆ ☆ ☆ ☆

ADDRESS:	Great Sand Dunes National Park and Preserve: Pinyon Flats Campground 11999 CO 150 Mosca, CO 81146
OPERATED BY:	National Park Service
INFORMATION:	(719) 378-2312; www.nps.gov/grsa
OPEN:	All year
SITES:	88
EACH SITE HAS:	Picnic table, fire grate, tent pad
ASSIGNMENT:	First come, first served; no reservation
REGISTRATION:	Camping permit required; self-registration on site
FACILITIES:	Water spigots, flush toilets, community sinks
PARKING:	At campsites only
FEE:	$14 per night
ELEVATION:	8,200 feet
RESTRICTIONS:	*Pets:* On leash only *Fires:* In fire grates only *Alcohol:* At campsite only *Vehicles:* 35 feet *Other:* 6 people maximum per site; 14-day stay limit

Each loop has two comfort stations with flush toilets, drinking water, and sinks for washing your dishes. Between Loop A and Loop B is a small campground store that is open between May and September. It offers typical camp supplies, such as ice, wood, and soda. If you run out of something, buy it here; otherwise, I suggest making a major supply run before you get to the dunes.

Pinyon Flats can fill on summer weekends. It is a little on the busy side during summer weekdays. However, from September to May, the campground is quiet and most campsites are available. Late spring and early fall are the best times to visit.

Have you ever climbed a 700-foot sand dune? Here's your chance. Take the half-mile Dunes Trail from the campground down to the dunes and start climbing. The loose sand and deceptive distances make it more challenging than it seems. This is one place where your footprints never last for long. Eighteen miles of more foot-friendly trails lace the park. Head north from the campground on the Little Medano Trail 1.2 miles to a cliff overlooking the dunes. The Pinyon Flats Trail connects the campground with the visitor center. The Wellington Ditch Trail is an easy hike along an old settler's irrigation flow. The high country awaits you on the Mosca Pass Trail.

In the summer, there are ranger-led walks every day and ranger programs every evening. Keep your camera handy at all times. The ever-changing light and dunes combine to present an evolving landscape as you explore the environment. These are the largest sand dunes in North America. The unexpected setting for them makes the Great Sand Dunes experience an eye-opening reward and very worth the stop.

Outside the park is the short walk to Zapata Falls. It is on public land a few miles south of the monument on Colorado 150. You can extend the hike 3 more miles up to alpine Zapata Lake. Nearby San Luis Lakes State Park offers fishing, boating, and wildlife viewing. Thousands of acres of the Sangre de Cristo Wilderness lie east of the dunes. A primitive road skirts the monument and heads into this vast national-forest land.

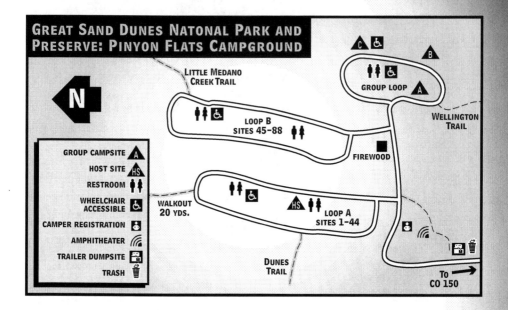

GREAT SAND DUNES NATONAL PARK AND PRESERVE: PINYON FLATS CAMPGROUND

N

LITTLE MEDANO CREEK TRAIL

GROUP LOOP

C

B

A

WELLINGTON TRAIL

LOOP B SITES 45–88

FIREWOOD

GROUP CAMPSITE A
HOST SITE HS
RESTROOM
WHEELCHAIR ACCESSIBLE
CAMPER REGISTRATION
AMPHITHEATER
TRAILER DUMPSITE
TRASH

WALKOUT 20 YDS.

HS

LOOP A SITES 1–44

DUNES TRAIL

To CO 150

GETTING THERE

From Blanca, drive west on US 160 for 5.2 miles to CO 150. Turn right on CO 150 and follow it for 16 miles to Great Sand Dunes National Monument.

GPS COORDINATES

UTM Zone (WGS84)	13S
Easting	0455530
Northing	4177790
Latitude	N 37° 44' 46.9"
Longitude	W 105° 30' 17"

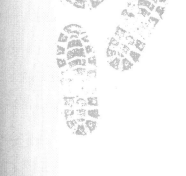

*Cool off in the
lake country of the
San Juan Mountains.*

SUMMER COMES LATE HIGH in the San Juan
Mountains. Mix Lake, at 10,000 feet, enjoys the
blessings and curses of a short season. It is
blessed with light use and a stunning high-country
landscape, but the season is short and the weather can
be rough. The campground is integrated into the varied topography and vegetation of the land. Mix Lake is
scenic itself, but so are other nearby lakes, Platoro
Reservoir, and the rugged South San Juan Wilderness.

After you pass the pay station, the gravel campground road begins to switchback upward toward Mix
Lake. As you turn, the first three campsites surprisingly
appear on your right in a clearing surrounded by
young aspen. These sites are fairly close together, but
offer good views of the Conejos River valley below.
Continue up the mountain and pass campsite 4, all by
itself. It has a good view as well as offering the most in
solitude. Campsite 5 is perched on a hill with even better views, but is very close to the road.

Then come to the first loop, set in a mixed bag of
brush, rocks, grass, and scattered trees. The campground host resides here. The loop enters a dense
conifer stand with campsites offering nearly complete
shade and privacy. The sites in the center of the loop
are more open. These sites and those at the end of the
loop avail views of the valley below and the mountains
above. Nearly all of the 12 campsites are spread far
from one another.

The second loop is the highest and closest to Mix
Lake. It also offers just about any combination of sun
and shade. There are five campsites here. The two
sites closest to the short trail to the lake are the most
heavily used. There is a water spigot at the beginning
of this loop.

Mother Nature did an excellent job of landscaping this campground. The combination of meadows,

RATINGS

Beauty: ☆ ☆ ☆
Privacy: ☆ ☆ ☆ ☆
Spaciousness: ☆ ☆ ☆
Quiet: ☆ ☆ ☆ ☆
Security: ☆ ☆ ☆ ☆
Cleanliness: ☆ ☆ ☆ ☆

boulders, trees, and views will satisfy even the pickiest tent camper. There are three vault toilets in this widespread campground. One is down the hill by the first three campsites; the other two are in the two main loops.

The long drive and nearby private resorts conspire to make this a quiet campground. Expect to find a site on all but the busiest summer weekends. Supplies can be had in the little village of Platoro just a mile down the hill. Expect to be gouged a bit when you buy them.

There are, however, many good things nearby, like Mix Lake itself. A short trail leaving the upper loop will take you to an overlook. Beyond is the massive Conejos Peak. Dark blue Mix Lake sits waiting below, with rainbow trout ready to match wits with you. Just a mile distant is the much larger Platoro Reservoir. This dammed lake is 700 acres in size and offers rainbow and brown trout. Just up toward Stunner Pass are Lily Lake and Kerr Lake. These are accessible from Forest Service Road 257.

There are three convenient trailheads leading into the remote South San Juan Wilderness. The weathering of volcanic rock over the ages by wind, water, and glaciers has left jagged peaks, alpine lakes, and towering forests. Rugged trails and the lack of 14,000-foot-high mountains keep the crowds away. Two trails enter the wilderness from FS 105. Take Trail 719 for the short, but steep, climb past Tobacco Lake on the way to Conejos Peak, 13,172 feet of rock offering unspoiled views of the wilderness and beyond. After climbing Conejos Peak you'll be glad it wasn't 14,000 feet. Head up to Bear Lake on Trail 721. Or take a trip to the Three Forks, where the headwaters of the Conejos River come together. This trail, 712, starts beyond Platoros Reservoir. The Continental Divide Trail runs 40 miles through the length of the wilderness. Below the wilderness, the Conejos River is a popular fishing destination itself. The river scenery has been recommended for wild and scenic designation. It is interspersed with private holdings, so be careful about where you wet your line.

KEY INFORMATION

ADDRESS:	Mix Lake Campground Conejos Peak Ranger District 15571 CR T-5 La Jara, CO 81140
OPERATED BY:	USDA Forest Service, Rio Grande National Forest
INFORMATION:	(719) 274-8971; www.fs.fed.us/r2/riogrande
OPEN:	Memorial Day–Labor Day
SITES:	22
EACH SITE HAS:	Tent pad, fire ring
ASSIGNMENT:	First come, first served; no reservation
REGISTRATION:	On site
FACILITIES:	Water spigot, vault toilets, trash pick-up
PARKING:	At campsites only
FEE:	$12 per night
ELEVATION:	10,000 feet
RESTRICTIONS:	*Pets:* On leash only *Fires:* In fire rings only *Alcohol:* At campsites only *Vehicles:* 25 feet *Other:* 14-day stay limit

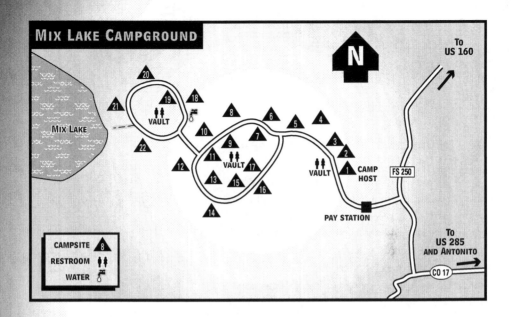

GETTING THERE

From Antonito drive 22 miles west on CO 17 to FS 250. Turn right on FS 250 for 24 miles to the signed left turn for Mix Lake Campground. Follow this road for 1 mile to Mix Lake Campground.

GPS COORDINATES

UTM Zone (WGS84)   13S
Easting   0363016
Northing   4135745
Latitude   N 37° 21' 29.8"
Longitude   W 106° 32' 48"

MANY CLAIM **MUELLER STATE PARK** to have views and scenery in Colorado second only to Rocky Mountain National Park. While this is debatable, it is evident that Mueller is blessed with a panoramic piece of land. Pikes Peak is in full view to the east and a long stretch of the Continental Divide lies in sight to the west. The immediate spruce, fir, and aspen slopes, broken with meadows and rock outcrops, serve as the canvas on which a clean, well-kept campground and a complete network of trails make up Mueller State Park.

The commendable upkeep of quality facilities is immediately noticeable when you arrive at Mueller. While riding the smooth, paved road to the immaculate, well-groomed campground, you'll wish all tenting locales could look this nice. The camping area is set in the high country along Revenuers Ridge, with several roads spurring off the main ridge road. The first spur road is Peak View. Here, five campsites are set in woods that look up to Pikes Peak. These sites are usually dominated by RVs and are among 11 total campsites that are open year-round.

The main campground road, divided into two one-way roads, has campsites all along it, including several pull-through sites. Then, Conifer Ridge splits off to the right. True to its name, spruce, fir, and pine cloak its slopes. All types of campers enjoy this area. Farther up Revenuers Ridge on your left is Prospectors Ridge. Here is a 12-site walk-in tent camping area. The woods are thick and campsites are strung out far from one another for more than 100 yards. If you want the maximum in solitude and privacy, pitch your tent here.

More campsites are laid out along the main road as you continue to Turkey Meadow. The meadow is a ten-site, walk-in tent camping area. Pine and fir trees shade most of the campsites, except those on the

> *Mueller is the ideal place to break into Rocky Mountain tent camping and hiking.*

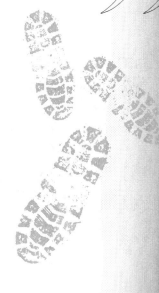

RATINGS

Beauty: ✿ ✿ ✿ ✿ ✿
Privacy: ✿ ✿ ✿
Spaciousness: ✿ ✿ ✿
Quiet: ✿ ✿ ✿
Security: ✿ ✿ ✿ ✿ ✿
Cleanliness: ✿ ✿ ✿ ✿ ✿

KEY INFORMATION

ADDRESS: Mueller State Park Campground
P.O. Box 39
Divide, CO 80814

OPERATED BY: Colorado State Parks

INFORMATION: (719) 687-2366;
parks.state.co.us

OPEN: Main campground mid-May–mid-October; Peak View Loop and 6 other sites all year

SITES: 22 walk-in tent-only sites, 110 other

EACH SITE HAS: Tent-only has tent pad, fire grate, picnic table; others also have water and electricity

ASSIGNMENT: By reservation, May 12–October 8) or pick an available site on arrival

REGISTRATION: (800) 678-CAMP (2267), (303) 470-1144 in Denver, or www.reserveamerica.com

FACILITIES: Hot showers, vault and flush toilets, laundry, phone

PARKING: At campsites or walk-in tent camping parking area

FEE: $5 Parks Pass plus $14 per night walk-in tent site, $18 others

ELEVATION: 9,500 feet

RESTRICTIONS: *Pets:* On leash only, not allowed on trails
Fires: In fire grates only
Alcohol: 3.2% beer only
Vehicles: 2 allowed at larger sites
Other: 14-day stay limit

meadow's edge; no matter where you are, the view of Pikes Peak is majestic. Feel fortunate if you get one of these campsites.

The campground ends with more campsites and an auto turnaround on Grouse Mountain. The tent camping areas are the best, but there is not a bad site in this well-designed campground. Water spigots and vault toilets are situated throughout Mueller. The showers, flush toilets, and laundry facilities are centrally located in the Camper Services building.

This campground stays booked from June through August. If you want to stay here—and I highly recommend that you do—come during the week, and make reservations no matter what time of year you camp. It is an ideal starter park for camping novices, and veterans will appreciate the extra special touch the state puts on at Mueller.

The same goes for recreation here. The trails are well marked and maintained. There are more than 85 miles of pathways, most open to both bikers and hikers of all skill levels. Some trails are also open to horseback riders. In the backcountry, you can hike to views, open meadows, and old homesteads and mines. There are several ponds in the backcountry for folks to fish. Four-Mile Creek offers stream fishing for trout.

The south end of Mueller has the Four-Mile Day Use Area. This is the trailhead for the popular hike up to Dome Rock. This trek involves several creek crossings. You may see some bighorn sheep from this rock, which rises 800 feet above the valley below.

Park personnel can steer you in the right direction for a trail of your ability. Go to the visitor center for answers to questions and also check out the indoor wildlife habitat there. Rangers lead nature programs during the summer in this wildlife-rich park of 12,000 acres. Mueller State Park can get you on your way to being a Rocky Mountain hiking and camping pro.

Also, while you are in the area, make a side trip to the mining town of Cripple Creek and Victor. The historic mining communities have been revamped, offering a little history and a lot of gaming.

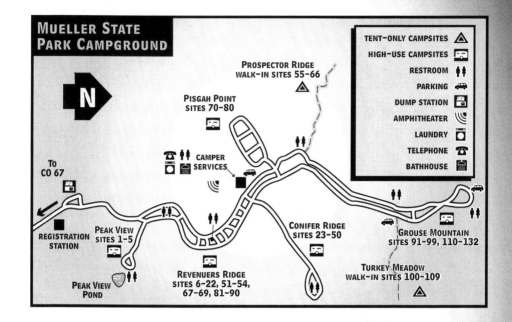

N

PROSPECTOR RIDGE
WALK-IN SITES 55-66

PISGAH POINT
SITES 70-80

TO
CO 67

CAMPER
SERVICES

REGISTRATION
STATION

PEAK VIEW
SITES 1-5

PEAK VIEW
POND

REVENUERS RIDGE
SITES 6-22, 51-54,
67-69, 81-90

CONIFER RIDGE
SITES 23-50

GROUSE MOUNTAIN
SITES 91-99, 110-132

TURKEY MEADOW
WALK-IN SITES 100-109

TENT-ONLY CAMPSITES
HIGH-USE CAMPSITES
RESTROOM
PARKING
DUMP STATION
AMPHITHEATER
LAUNDRY
TELEPHONE
BATHHOUSE

GETTING THERE

From Woodland Park, drive west on CO 24 for 7 miles to Divide. Then turn left on CO 67 south for 3.5 miles to Mueller State Park, which will be on your right.

GPS COORDINATES

UTM Zone (WGS84)	13S
Easting	0485930
Northing	4305840
Latitude	N 38° 54' 5.9"
Longitude	W 105° 9' 43"

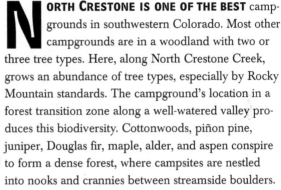

> *North Crestone offers creekside camping in a riparian forest perched against the Sangre de Cristo Mountains.*

NORTH **C**RESTONE **IS ONE OF THE BEST** campgrounds in southwestern Colorado. Most other campgrounds are in a woodland with two or three tree types. Here, along North Crestone Creek, grows an abundance of tree types, especially by Rocky Mountain standards. The campground's location in a forest transition zone along a well-watered valley produces this biodiversity. Cottonwoods, piñon pine, juniper, Douglas fir, maple, alder, and aspen conspire to form a dense forest, where campsites are nestled into nooks and crannies between streamside boulders.

Being in the foothills of the Sangre de Cristo Mountains contributes to making this a desirable place to tent camp. Craggy, barren, snow-covered peaks, alpine lakes, far-reaching views of the San Luis Valley and mountains beyond make the hiking some of the most scenic in the state. The upper reaches of these highlands are protected wilderness.

The campground begins just after you enter the Rio Grande National Forest. On your left is a rocky, tree-studded canyon wall. To your right is the crashing Crestone Creek, shaded by all those wonderful trees. A heavy understory of younger trees and alder screens you from everyone else.

The first set of campsites are set into the woods. The camper parking spots are along the two-way road. At each site, the picnic tables and fire grates are located a short walk from the parking spots closer to the creek. A vault toilet and pump well serve these campsites.

The next set of campsites are farther up the road by a good 100 yards. These campsites are notched into flat areas among the boulders and trees wherever they can fit. There are a couple of sites that offer some sun, but expect to be in the shade most of the time in this valley environment.

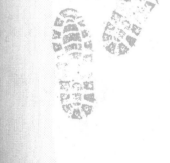

RATINGS

Beauty: ✿ ✿ ✿ ✿ ✿
Privacy: ✿ ✿ ✿ ✿ ✿
Spaciousness: ✿ ✿ ✿
Quiet: ✿ ✿ ✿ ✿
Security: ✿ ✿ ✿
Cleanliness: ✿ ✿ ✿ ✿

The final set of two campsites is located just before the end of the road and trailhead parking. One campsite is across the road from the creek—it's the only one that isn't directly next to North Crestone Creek. There is a new vault toilet and pump well up here. A vehicle turnaround and the mountains lie beyond the last campsites.

This is a popular weekend campground, being so beautiful and having so few sites. The upside of having only 13 sites is that even when it's busy, it doesn't seem crowded. But if you want to camp here on a weekend, try to get here on Friday night or early Saturday morning. You won't regret losing a little sleep to camp at North Crestone.

The Sangre de Cristo Wilderness is just a walk away from your tent. The North Crestone Creek Trail leaves the upper end of the campground, heads up, and connects to other trails in the wilderness, enabling trips to the high country. Venable Pass is 5 miles distant, as is North Crestone Lake. The trails here are well marked and maintained. You can fish the creek, which tumbles as waterfalls much of the distance, or North Crestone Lake, where the fishing is said to be good. Wildlife-viewing possibilities include seeing bighorn sheep and bears. Speaking of bears, they are known to slip into the campground during lean years, so store your food properly.

Campers sometimes walk the mile to the hamlet of Crestone. Here they have a small general store, a tavern, and an eatery. The living is nice and slow here. No tourist traps, just nice people. While you are down there, check out a few more hiking opportunities.

If you take the road past the post office in tiny Crestone and follow it 2 miles up, you will come to the South Crestone and Willow Lake Trails. South Crestone climbs a few miles to South Crestone Lake. The Willow Lake Trail is 3 miles to Willow Lake and Willow Falls. This whole country is very photographer-friendly. I believe the Sangre de Cristos are the most scenic mountains in Colorado. Come here and rate them for yourself.

KEY INFORMATION

ADDRESS:	North Crestone Creek Campground Saguache Ranger District 46525 CO 114 Saguache, CO 81149
OPERATED BY:	USDA Forest Service
INFORMATION:	(719) 655-2547; www.fs.fed.us/r2/ riogrande
OPEN:	Memorial Day– Labor Day
SITES:	13
EACH SITE HAS:	Picnic table, fire ring
ASSIGNMENT:	First come, first served; no reservation
REGISTRATION:	Self-registration on site
FACILITIES:	Pump well water, vault toilets, trash pick-up
PARKING:	At campsites only
FEE:	$9 per night
ELEVATION:	8,300 feet
RESTRICTIONS:	*Pets:* On leash only *Fires:* In fire grates only *Alcohol:* At campsites only *Vehicles:* 25 feet *Other:* 14-day stay limit

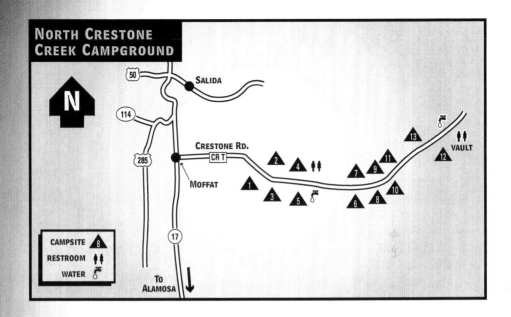

North Crestone Creek Campground

GETTING THERE

From Moffat, drive east on CR T (Crestone Road) for 13 miles to the hamlet of Crestone. Follow CR T for 1.2 miles until it turns into FS 950. North Crestone will be on your right.

GPS COORDINATES

UTM Zone (WGS84)   13S
Easting   0439460
Northing   4207800
Latitude   N 38° 0' 57.8"
Longitude   W 105° 41' 21"

TRUJILLO MEADOWS CAMPGROUND

TRUJILLO **M**EADOWS **EXUDES** a high-mountain aura from its perch near Cumbres Pass and the New Mexico state line. Thick stands of conifers yield to open clearings of grass where cool breezes make summer wildflowers sway back and forth against the backdrop of the San Juan Mountains. The campground is spread wide over the montane setting, standing at 10,000 feet, making the 49-site getaway a much more intimate spot. Trujillo Meadows Reservoir is an attractive mountain impoundment that anglers and canoers can enjoy. The historic Cumbres and Toltec Railroad chugs through Cumbres Pass, offering scenic tours between Chama, New Mexico, and Antonito, Colorado. Possibly the most remote and rugged wilderness in Colorado, the South San Juan Wilderness is only a few miles away. There, hikers have an opportunity to get back to the Colorado that the Indians knew.

Leave the well-maintained FS 118 and enter Trujillo Meadows. Pass the campground host, located at the entrance for your safety. The upper loop, starting with campsite 1, is much more open. The campsites are set among forest and meadow, giving campers many site, shade, and privacy options. A sunny site may be a good choice on a cool, early summer day.

The second loop, starting with campsite 16, has many tent camping sites, but also has pull-through campsites that will attract the big rigs. Whoever camps here will enjoy good mountain views, as much of this campsite is in open meadowland with only occasional tree cover. Another small loop spurs off this loop but is often closed unless the campground is full.

Keep forward and enter the lower portion of the campground. Here you will find campsites 25 through 49 in an ultradense spruce and fir woodland, which gives off those evergreen aromas that I associate with the high country. This loop slopes off toward a small

> *This is one of the more scenic and well-kept campgrounds in the Rio Grande National Forest, with much to see and do nearby.*

RATINGS

Beauty: ✪ ✪ ✪ ✪
Privacy: ✪ ✪ ✪ ✪
Spaciousness: ✪ ✪ ✪ ✪
Quiet: ✪ ✪ ✪
Security: ✪ ✪ ✪ ✪ ✪
Cleanliness: ✪ ✪ ✪ ✪

ADDRESS: Trujillo Meadows
Campground
Conejos Peak
Ranger District
15571 CR T-5
La Jara, CO 81140

OPERATED BY: USDA Forest
Service, Rio Grande
National Forest

INFORMATION: (719) 274-8971;
www.fs.fed.us/r2/
riogrande

OPEN: Memorial Day–
Labor Day

SITES: 49

EACH SITE HAS: Picnic table, fire
grate

ASSIGNMENT: First come,
first served;
no reservation

REGISTRATION: On site

FACILITIES: Water spigots, vault
toilet

PARKING: At campsites only

FEE: $14 per night

ELEVATION: 10,100 feet

RESTRICTIONS: *Pets:* On leash only
Fires: In fire grates
only
Alcohol: At campsites
only
Vehicles: 25 feet
Other: 14-day stay
limit

canyon lying off to the right. The sites here are fairly close together, but the crowded forest eliminates privacy issues, actually making this the campground's most private loop.

Save your walking for the wilderness trails here, as bathrooms and water spigots are spread evenly throughout the campground. Expect Trujillo Meadows to fill on holidays and weekends in the later summer. Get your supplies in the surrounding lowlands; stores are very scarce in the San Juans.

Trujillo Meadow Reservoir lies just a short distance from the campground. Anglers can cast their line for trout. If you bring a boat, keep your large motors home, this reservoir is wakeless. A canoe would be a better watercraft choice.

Hikers need trails to walk! And the South San Juan Wilderness is as wild as Colorado gets and has more than 180 miles of trails to tramp. The last known grizzly bear in the state was killed here in 1979; many folks think if there are grizzlies left anywhere in Colorado, it will be here in the South San Juans. This place is rugged. Pick up the Continental Divide Trail at Cumbres Pass and head north into the South San Juan Wilderness. For closer wilderness access, take FS 1C to the upper Los Piños River trailhead (you passed it on FS 118 to the campground). Take Trail 736 and enter an alpine land of jagged mountains and sparkling lakes. Other trails spur off Colorado 7 on the way up from Antonito. Take Trail 733 up to Red Lake.

For a less sweaty way to see the scenery, take the Cumbres and Toltec Scenic Railroad. Ride in an open-air car, pulled by a coal-burning locomotive, and get an eyeful of mountainous border country. It was originally built in the 1870s to access the mining fields of the Silverton area. The Cumbres and Toltec Railroad is now listed on the National Register of Historic Places. So climb aboard, and let those old-time engines do all the work.

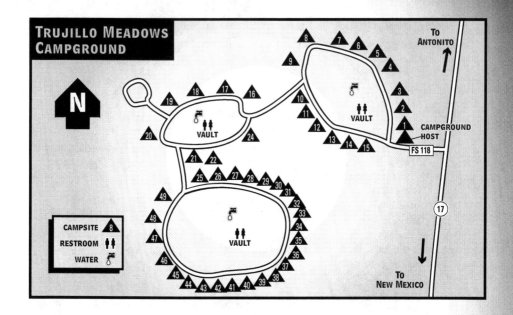

N

To
ANTONITO

CAMPGROUND
HOST

FS 118

VAULT

VAULT

VAULT

17

To
NEW MEXICO

CAMPSITE 8
RESTROOM
WATER

GETTING THERE

From Antonito drive 37
miles west on CO 17 to FS
118. Turn right on FS 118
and follow it 2 miles to Trujillo Meadows Campground,
which will be on your right.

GPS COORDINATES

UTM Zone (WGS84)	13S
Easting	0371130
Northing	4101030
Latitude	N 37° 2' 48.3"
Longitude	W 106° 26' 55"

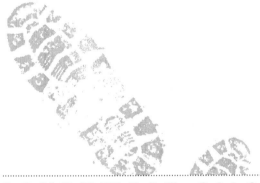

SOUTHWEST COLORADO

39
BLACK CANYON OF THE GUNNISON NATIONAL PARK: NORTH RIM CAMPGROUND

YOU WON'T BELIEVE WHAT A DEEP and narrow gorge the Black Canyon is until you actually see it. There are many places to access the gorge, but the North Rim is the best. It is the most quiet and boasts the better campground in the park, set on the rim's edge in an ancient piñon–juniper forest. Instead of looking up at snowy mountains—your typical Colorado view—you will be looking down into a nearly 2,000-foot-deep canyon. Views can be had by hiking or by a scenic drive. You can hike along the rim or drop down into the gorge itself, where the fishing is great along a stretch of Colorado's Gold Medal Waters. The best climbing in the state can be done here at "The Black," as it's known in the climbing world.

Make your drive from Crawford and slightly descend to the canyon along Grizzly Gulch. Turn right, pass the Ranger Station, and come to the North Rim Campground. Enter the loop and the piñon–juniper forest, which is complemented with Gambel oak and the bird-attracting serviceberry. As you look for a campsite, note the gnarled trees here. Some are more than 700 years old! It is a rare opportunity indeed to camp among such ancient trees.

The campground lies on a fair slope heading down toward the canyon. The smaller gorge of SOB Draw (which is short for what you think it is) wraps around the campground. Campsites are on both sides of the road beneath the old trees, which offer the ideal amount of sun and shade. The understory is primarily dirt, which can make for a dusty campsite. Overall, the campsites are on the small side, which discourages nearly all but tent campers, especially after big rig drivers see how the old trees crowd the road. They just turn right around. A vault toilet and water spigot are in the center of the small campground. Be advised that the water may not be turned on early or late in the camping season.

> *The North Rim Campground is a rock climber's mecca. If you don't climb, come here anyway; there are other ways to enjoy the gorgeous scenery.*

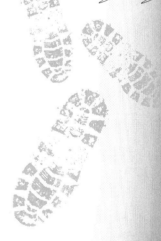

RATINGS

Beauty: ☆ ☆ ☆ ☆
Privacy: ☆ ☆ ☆
Spaciousness: ☆ ☆ ☆
Quiet: ☆ ☆ ☆ ☆
Security: ☆ ☆ ☆ ☆ ☆
Cleanliness: ☆ ☆ ☆ ☆

ADDRESS:	**North Rim Campground 102 Elk Creek Gunnison, CO 81230**
OPERATED BY:	**National Park Service**
INFORMATION:	**(970) 641-2337; www.nps.gov/blca**
OPEN:	**Mid-May– mid-October**
SITES:	**13**
EACH SITE HAS:	**Picnic table, fire grate**
ASSIGNMENT:	**First come, first served; no reservation**
REGISTRATION:	**Self-registration on site**
FACILITIES:	**Water spigot, vault toilet**
PARKING:	**At campsites only**
FEE:	**$12 per night; $7 park pass per vehicle**
ELEVATION:	**7,700 feet**
RESTRICTIONS:	*Pets:* **On leash only** *Fires:* **In fire grates only** *Alcohol:* **At campsites only** *Vehicles:* **26 feet** *Other:* **14-day stay limit**

At the end of the loop is the Chasm View Trail. During my visit with a friendly ranger, he raved about this trail. I just had to hike it first thing. Even after the hype, the view into the gorge was simply unbelievable. It is so narrow and deep! The Gunnison River emits its roar, but it is fairly faint up here. There are old trees on the Chasm View Trail too. It made me want to hit the other views in the park.

The North Vista Trail leaves from the ranger station. The path goes along the North Rim of the Gunnison to a high point on a nearby ridge. There are views into SOB Draw. But the highlight is the side trip to Exclamation Point. And as the ranger stated, "They call it Exclamation Point for a reason." Some of the best views of the inner canyon are found here.

So you want to make the challenging descent to, and more challenging ascent from, the canyon floor? There are three ways in from the North Rim. The SOB Draw Route starts near the campground. It is two hours down and four hours up the 2-mile route. Watch for the poison ivy growing thick along the way. Long Draw is a mile-long drop that starts near the Balanced Rock Overlook; beware of poison ivy growing 5 feet high here. Slide Draw is very steep and starts near the Kneeling Camel View. Anglers in search of the big trout can brave the poison ivy and test the lesser-fished waters.

There are views along the 5-mile gravel road where you can tour the North Rim by car. Simply leave the campground and keep driving along the rim. Be very careful—the views are quite distracting. At the end of this road is the Deadhorse Trail. This 2.5-mile path traces an old road past springs and provides views into Deadhorse Gulch and the main canyon.

The ranger on duty near the campground is often a climbing ranger. The ranger has a route book for climbers to consult and will assist you in choosing routes. Inexperienced climbers should first go with other climbers or stick to the trails. All climbers and backcountry visitors must obtain a free backcountry permit at the ranger station.

The Black Canyon of the Gunnison is a unique physical feature of Colorado and is a must-see for both natives and tourists.

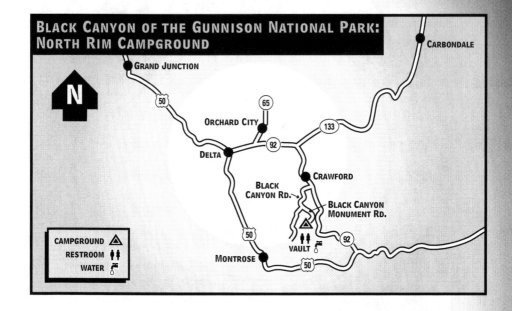

CARBONDALE

GRAND JUNCTION

N

50

65

ORCHARD CITY

133

92

DELTA

CRAWFORD

BLACK CANYON RD.

BLACK CANYON MONUMENT RD.

CAMPGROUND

RESTROOM

WATER

50

VAULT

92

MONTROSE

50

GETTING THERE

From Crawford, drive south on CO 92 for 3 miles to Black Canyon Road. Turn right on Black Canyon Road and follow it as it twists and turns through the countryside for 6 miles to Black Canyon Monument Road. Turn left on Black Canyon Monument Road and follow it for 5 more miles to the monument. Once at the monument, turn right at the first intersection to access the North Rim Campground, just a short distance away.

GPS COORDINATES

UTM Zone (WGS84)	13S
Easting	0253590
Northing	4296990
Latitude	N 38° 47' 14.3"
Longitude	W 107° 50' 15"

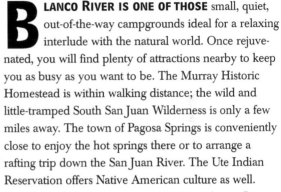

> *Blanco River*
> *Campground makes*
> *a great base camp*
> *for exploring the South*
> *San Juan Mountains.*

BLANCO **R**IVER **IS ONE OF THOSE** small, quiet, out-of-the-way campgrounds ideal for a relaxing interlude with the natural world. Once rejuvenated, you will find plenty of attractions nearby to keep you as busy as you want to be. The Murray Historic Homestead is within walking distance; the wild and little-tramped South San Juan Wilderness is only a few miles away. The town of Pagosa Springs is conveniently close to enjoy the hot springs there or to arrange a rafting trip down the San Juan River. The Ute Indian Reservation offers Native American culture as well.

Blanco River campground is situated on a flat beside the gurgling Blanco River. Pass the picnic area and enter the loop. To your right is a steep hill covered in Douglas fir. A grassy meadow punctuated with large narrow-leaf cottonwoods occupies the center of the loop, as do the first two campsites. Each one is placed near the shade of a cottonwood. These spacious campsites look little used, maybe due to the apparent lack of privacy. But campsite privacy is not much of an issue at this underused campground because each campsite is spread far from its neighbor.

The dirt road loops around where the steep hill meets the Blanco River. Here is the third campsite, right by the river, beneath a large ponderosa pine. You can access the river easily after making your way past a fence, which keeps cows from camping with you. The fourth campsite is beneath large ponderosa pines too.

The fifth campsite is the most popular. It drops off the flat down by the river in a grove of fir. You can get sun by the river, yet enjoy shade whenever the sun gets too strong. The sixth campsite is at the end of the loop and enjoys morning shade. It is also by the set of vault toilets for each gender. The pump well is back 200 feet toward the picnic area. It'll give your arm a

RATINGS

Beauty: ☆ ☆ ☆
Privacy: ☆ ☆ ☆ ☆
Spaciousness: ☆ ☆ ☆ ☆ ☆
Quiet: ☆ ☆ ☆ ☆ ☆
Security: ☆ ☆ ☆
Cleanliness: ☆ ☆ ☆ ☆

workout, so be prepared to pump a while before that tasty water comes out.

Don't be surprised if you are the lone camper here. It should never fill up except on the busiest summer holiday. I stayed with one other group on a Sunday night in mid-June. That same group had Blanco River all to themselves the previous Saturday night!

A French Canadian named Provencher thought this area was a fine place as well. He had a homestead and sawmill up the Blanco River around 1900. But he was flooded out and moved up the hill in 1913. You can follow the old road from the picnic area that leads to the site. Here you'll find the remains of the original barn, a hand-hewn log cabin, and a corral in a meadow with a view deep into the San Juans. The property changed hands over the years until the Forest Service took it over in 1970.

The volcanic rock of the South San Juan Wilderness has eroded into excellent soil and nurtures some of the finest forests in the Rockies. Glaciers have carved deep valleys and ragged peaks, making these mountains ideal for photographers. This wild land harbored the last known grizzly bears in Colorado. Some believe they may be here still. Don't let that possibility scare you, for there is too much beauty to be seen.

Blanco Basin Road offers good access to the South San Juan Wilderness. From here you can walk the upper reaches of the Blanco River. Bring your rod along if you head up Fish Creek or Fish Lake. It's a short walk to Opal Lake, which is named for the milky color of its waters. Fishing for trout is good in the Blanco River right from the campground as well.

The V Rock trailhead on FS 663 south of Blanco River offers access to Buckles Lake, the upper Navajo River basin, and the Spring Creek Lakes. Nearby Eight Mile Mesa is a featured mountain-biking area and sports a lookout tower that offers a view of the Pagosa country.

After all that hiking and biking, you need to relax in a hot spring. Drive into Pagosa Springs and enjoy the naturally hot waters beside the San Juan River at The Springs. Different pools are different temperatures—see how much heat you can take. The mineral-rich springs range from 94°F to 111°F.

KEY INFORMATION

ADDRESS:	Blanco River Campground Pagosa Ranger District 108 Second Street Pagosa Springs, CO 81147
OPERATED BY:	USDA Forest Service, San Juan National Forest
INFORMATION:	(970) 264-2268; www.fs.fed.us/r2/sanjuan
OPEN:	Mid-May–mid-November
SITES:	6
EACH SITE HAS:	Fire ring, picnic table
ASSIGNMENT:	First come, first served; no reservation
REGISTRATION:	Self-registration on site
FACILITIES:	Pump well, vault toilets, trash pick-up
PARKING:	At campsites only
FEE:	$10 per night
ELEVATION:	7,200 feet
RESTRICTIONS:	*Pets:* On leash only *Fires:* In fire rings only *Alcohol:* At campsites only *Vehicles:* 35 feet *Other:* 14-day stay limit

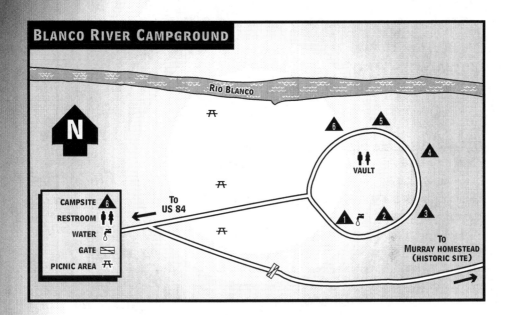

GETTING THERE

From Pagosa Springs, drive south on US 84 for 10.2 miles to FS 656. You will cross the Rio Blanco and then the Blanco River on bridges. After the second river crossing, turn left on FS 656 and follow it 2.5 miles to Blanco River campground.

You can also set up a rafting trip down the San Juan. Outfitters are located all around town. A typical trip will take you down the varied rapids. Other trips offer trout fishing. Pagosa Springs is a western town that hasn't been taken over by big-bucks development and is a pleasure to visit.

GPS COORDINATES

UTM Zone (WGS84)   13S
Easting   0332770
Northing   4112600
Latitude   N 37° 8' 40.9"
Longitude   W 106° 52' 58"

41
BURRO BRIDGE
CAMPGROUND

YOU'VE HEARD THE SAYING BEFORE about real estate—the three most important things are location, location, location. Location is indeed the best thing about Burro Bridge. The site of the small campground is the head of a meadow, fringed in woodland on a perch above the West Dolores River. It meets the expectations of high-country beauty you've come to expect in Colorado's national-forest campgrounds. However, the nearby Lizard Head Wilderness exceeds the beauty expected from the state's wilderness areas. The state's westernmost fourteener and views of the arid, red rock country to the west are two highlights of this wilderness. And proximity to the Lizard Head makes Burro Bridge a tent camper's choice campground. Tent campers with horses are welcome here too.

The 14 campsites are strung along a two-way gravel road with a vehicle turnaround at the end. Aspen and spruce are the primary forest components. The understory is grass, flowers, and young aspen. To your left are the meadow and a rising mountain of solid aspen. To your right is the small canyon of the West Dolores River. An attractive log fence borders the campground along the edge of the precipice that drops down into the West Dolores River. (The Forest Service doesn't want you to fall into the river on a midnight bathroom run.)

The first campsite is nestled in a shade-lending spruce coppice. The next two are by the canyon, but are more open and each has a shade tree near the picnic table. Farther down, a few sites are away from the river in the sunny meadow. This affords little shade, but good views of the surrounding mountains.

The road climbs gently up along the meadow, passing the vault toilets for each gender, a pump well, and a small horse corral. Campsites continue on both sides of the road, sunny sites on the left and shadier

> *Burro Bridge is next to the Lizard Head Wilderness, which encompasses the high peaks of the San Miguel Mountains.*

RATINGS

Beauty: ✩ ✩ ✩
Privacy: ✩ ✩ ✩
Spaciousness: ✩ ✩ ✩ ✩ ✩
Quiet: ✩ ✩ ✩ ✩
Security: ✩ ✩ ✩
Cleanliness: ✩ ✩ ✩

KEY INFORMATION

ADDRESS: Burro Bridge
Campground
Mancos-Dolores
Ranger District
100 North Sixth
Street
Dolores, CO 81323

OPERATED BY: USDA Forest
Service, San Juan
National Forest

INFORMATION: (970) 882-7296;
www.fs.fed.us/r2/
sanjuan

OPEN: June–September

SITES: 14

EACH SITE HAS: Picnic table, fire ring

ASSIGNMENT: First come,
first served;
no reservation

REGISTRATION: Self-registration on
site

FACILITIES: Pump well water,
vault toilets, trash
pick-up, horse
corrals ($5 per day)

PARKING: At campsites only

FEE: $12 per night

ELEVATION: 9,000 feet

RESTRICTIONS: *Pets:* On leash only
Fires: In fire rings
only
Alcohol: At campsites
only
Vehicles: 35 feet
Other: 14-day stay
limit

sites on the right. There is a campsite surrounded by young aspen in the middle of the vehicle turnaround.

The last three sites on the outer auto turnaround are beneath a thick stand of spruce and are very shady. The last campsite is set far from the road and is Burro Bridge's most private site. Overall, the large distance between campsites makes privacy less of an issue and abundant site spaciousness the norm.

With so many campgrounds in the area and being farther from the main roads, Burro Bridge receives light use. You may have it all to yourself on a weekday. Weekends may see a few other tent and horse campers, but expect to find a campsite on all but the major summer holidays.

Though it is not the highest peak, the 400-foot spire at its top makes Lizard Head the most conspicuous mountain in the wilderness. It is not scalable except by expert climbers. There are three fourteeners (Colorado-speak for 14,000-foot or higher mountains) in the Lizard Head. Alpine lakes, waterfalls, and deserted mines complement the high mountains.

Your ticket to all this is the Navajo Lake Trail, which starts a mile above Burro Bridge. The trail crosses the West Dolores, passes two sets of falls, then comes to Navajo Lake. Much of this hiking will be at or above the timber line, so bring clothing for foul weather. A good loop hike uses Navajo Lake Trail then returns to the road above Burro Bridge on the Kilpacker Trail. A little of this hike will be on a forest road.

A good view of the peaks of Lizard Head can be seen while driving over to Colorado 145 to Lizard Head Pass. The historic Rio Grande Southern Railroad wound through this pass. Start a high-country hike from Lizard Head Pass to the spire of Lizard Head on the Lizard Head Trail.

The Calico Trail is also nearby Burro Bridge. Use Forest Service Road 471 to make this 17-mile network of trails any length you like. Mountain bikers should take note of the Stoner Mesa area. This and the Taylor Mesa area offer 150 square miles of high-country forest for hikers, bikers, horse riders, and four-wheel-drive vehicles. Set up camp at Burro Bridge, get out your San Juan National Forest map, and begin exploring.

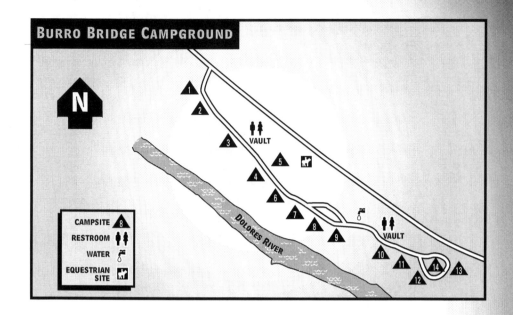

BURRO BRIDGE CAMPGROUND

N

VAULT

DOLORES RIVER

VAULT

CAMPSITE 8
RESTROOM
WATER
EQUESTRIAN
SITE

GETTING THERE

From Dolores, drive north
on CO 145 for 13 miles, then
turn left on FS 535 (West
Dolores Road). Follow FS
535 for 25 miles to Burro
Bridge Campground, which
will be on your right.

GPS COORDINATES

UTM Zone (WGS84)	12S
Easting	0758410
Northing	4186030
Latitude	N 37° 47' 6.3"
Longitude	W 108° 3' 56"

> *The camping here is free, quiet, and relaxed.*

AS YOU PULL INTO CATHEDRAL ROCK and look for a campsite, you begin to wonder why the Forest Service doesn't charge you to camp here. Then you pat your wallet, dismiss the thought, and go about the business of choosing a spot to pitch your tent. And there are plenty of good campsites in this campground, set in a mixed forest of aspen and blue spruce along Embargo Creek. Cathedral Rock and the La Garita Mountains loom over the locale from across the creek.

The 29 campsites are split about evenly on two loops. The left-hand loop is higher up along the creek. In fact, the upper part of this loop lies astride the confluence of Embargo and Cathedral creeks. A small clearing lies in the lower center of the loop, as campsites are strung along the heavily wooded banks of Embargo Creek. The forest here is so dense that many of the campsites receive almost no sunlight at all. Others are more open as the loop enters a pocket of old aspens. Then the loop turns back downstream and comes to the clearing again. There is a little rock, Engelmann spruce, and ground juniper thrown into the forest mix. Vault toilets are located at each end of the loop for easy access.

The right-hand loop drops down along Embargo Creek. The woods are denser throughout this loop with very few sunny sites. Judging by the vegetation growing on some of the vehicle pull-in areas on the upper part of the loop, these sites receive very little use. The lower sites along the creek, though, get taken first (and taken they were on my visit). Three of the campsites were occupied by families that had been coming here for years; the trip to Cathedral was a sort of summer pilgrimage for them. They lauded the attributes of Cathedral until they found out it was going to be included in a campground guidebook, then

RATINGS

Beauty: ✩ ✩ ✩ ✩
Privacy: ✩ ✩ ✩
Spaciousness: ✩ ✩ ✩
Quiet: ✩ ✩ ✩ ✩
Security: ✩ ✩
Cleanliness: ✩ ✩ ✩

about-faced and made Cathedral sound like a mosquito-infested hole. Well, it is neither heaven nor hell for tent campers, but it is a nice slice of forest in which to relax and escape the trials of modern life. Cathedral is rarely more than half full—usually less than that—and it is very quiet. It fills maybe one or two weekends per season. The woods provide ample privacy, and the sites are average in size. It does have a worn-in look, like an old, comfortable shoe. This shoe will fit most tent campers.

Relaxing and getting away from it all are at the top of the list here. But if you get tent fever, there are some good hiking trails that leave right from the campground, and other trails are nearby. The Cathedral Creek Trail starts near campsite 1 and leads up Cathedral Creek to the Cathedral Rock. In early summer, wildflowers line the trail. Later in the summer you'll be eating strawberries and gooseberries. There are many crossings of the creek, eventually passing a waterfall on the way up to the jagged cliffs of Cathedral Rock.

The Embargo Creek Trail leaves the upper loop and heads toward Mesa Mountain along Embargo Creek. Views open up a few miles from the campground. The Fremont Camp Trail starts up Forest Service Road 640 a short piece above the campground. Here is where explorer John Fremont and his men spent a long and deadly winter.

Both Cathedral and Embargo creeks offer excellent trout fishing near the campground. Fly-fishing is easier below the campground in the lower elevations along Embargo Creek, where the forest is more open. But if you want to go for the big ones, head down to the Rio Grande. Many portions of the river are Colorado gold-medal fishing waters, which are catch-and-release areas, allowing the trout to grow larger. Rafting is also a popular way to enjoy the Rio Grande. The rapids are generally Class II and III. Outfitters are stationed in both South Fork and Del Norte.

KEY INFORMATION

ADDRESS: Cathedral Campground Divide Ranger District 13308 West US 160 Del Norte, CO 81132

OPERATED BY: USDA Forest Service, Rio Grande National Forest

INFORMATION: (719) 657-3321; www.fs.fed.us/r2/riogrande

OPEN: Memorial Day–Labor Day

SITES: 29

EACH SITE HAS: Picnic table, fire grates

ASSIGNMENT: First come, first served; no reservation

REGISTRATION: No registration

FACILITIES: Bring your own water; vault toilets

PARKING: At campsites only

FEE: No fee

ELEVATION: 9,400 feet

RESTRICTIONS: *Pets:* On leash only
Fires: In fire grates only
Alcohol: At campsites only
Vehicles: 35 feet
Other: 14-day stay limit

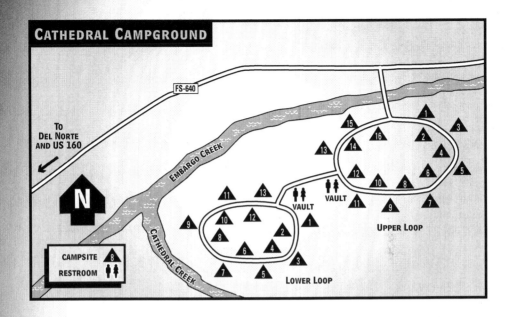

GETTING THERE

From Del Norte, head west on US 160 for 9 miles to Embargo Creek Road. Turn right on Embargo Creek Road and follow the signs for Cathedral Campground 15 miles distant on FS 650 then FS 640. Cathedral Campground will be on your right.

GPS COORDINATES

UTM Zone (WGS84)   13S
Easting   0358780
Northing   4187420
Latitude   N 37° 49' 24.1"
Longitude   W 106° 36' 16"

43
LOST LAKE
CAMPGROUND

THE SETTING AT **L**OST **L**AKE **C**AMPGROUND is classic. A shimmering jewel of water is perched high in the mountains with a forested backdrop, from which snowy, granite twin peaks rise majestically. Most of the campsites have views of this inspiring sight, as if the Kebler Pass Road wasn't scenic enough on the way up to Lost Lake. Rising out of the West Elk Wilderness, East Beckwith and West Beckwith mountains form twin sentinels over Lost Lake Slough, the body of water beside which you camp. The actual Lost Lake is farther up in the mountains, less than a mile distant.

Not only do you have some of the most scenic tent camping in Colorado, you are also within a mile of two wilderness areas: the West Elk and the Raggeds Wilderness to your north, which were those pointed peaks off to your left as you drove up. So if you get bored with relaxing and fishing at Lost Lake, there are nearly 300 miles of trails between the two wilderness areas on which to exhaust yourself.

When you finally make it to Lost Lake Slough, veer left; to your right are some Forest Service–owned cabins. No need to register or pay, the camping here is free. The main drive runs along the lake, and the first two campsites are large and have popular lake views. Then pass the pump well, which probably won't be working; bring your own water. Next are a few campsites that are directly lakeside on some less-than-level terrain. The view from here, however, may be worth a sloping night in the tent.

Beyond this, come to the campground drive, which leads away from the lake onto a hill wooded with conifers. The shade is welcome here on those relentless summer days, and the privacy is enhanced by the trees; however, your view of the mountains and lake is obstructed. A small meadow slopes off the drive at the turnaround. You pass one campsite in the center

> *The view is so good here that the Forest Service should charge a fee instead of letting you camp free.*

RATINGS

Beauty: ✩ ✩ ✩ ✩ ✩
Privacy: ✩ ✩ ✩
Spaciousness: ✩ ✩ ✩
Quiet: ✩ ✩ ✩ ✩
Security: ✩ ✩ ✩
Cleanliness: ✩ ✩ ✩

ADDRESS: Lost Lake
Campground
Paonia Ranger
District
P.O. Box 1030
North Rio Grande
Avenue
Paonia, CO 81428

OPERATED BY: USDA Forest
Service, Grand
Mesa, Uncompahgre
and Gunnison
National Forests

INFORMATION: (970) 527-4131;
www.fs.fed.us/r2/
gmug

OPEN: Mid-May–
mid-November

SITES: 11

EACH SITE HAS: Picnic table, fire
grate

ASSIGNMENT: First come,
first served;
no reservation

REGISTRATION: No registration

FACILITIES: Vault toilets (no
water)

PARKING: At campsites only

FEE: $10 per night

ELEVATION: 9,600 feet

RESTRICTIONS: *Pets:* On leash only
Fires: In fire grates
only
Alcohol: At campsites
only
Vehicles: 16 feet
Other: 14-day stay
limit

of the turnaround that is convenient to the vault toilet and one more campsite downslope in the woods opposite the lake. This last campsite is generally the last to be taken.

In the summer, Lost Lake will fill up on weekends. Earlier in the season, the weather can be chancy here. As always, call ahead before making the long drive to camp here or anywhere. The campground opening is dependent on the snow up here. The Forest Service will open the campground as soon as the road is open. If the campground is open, you should have no trouble finding a campsite on a weekday.

The serrated, prominent spires of the Ruby Range give the Raggeds Wilderness its name. Aspens and conifers grace the lower, wooded slopes. Trails lead into this land off Kebler Pass Road, both before and after the turnoff to Lost Lake Campground. On your way up, you passed the trailhead for Trail 836, which leads down Trout Creek. To enjoy the higher alpine country, drive toward Kebler Pass and head north on Trail 830, which passes a few lakes as it runs parallel to the Ruby Range.

A short walk away from the campgrounds is the Beckwith Pass Trail, which heads south into the 17,600-acre West Elk Wilderness. Your hike leads south to Beckwith Pass, which isn't usually passable until mid-July. It is a little more than 2 miles to the pass. From there, you can split left to the Cliff Creek Trail, which is actually just before the pass, or continue into the heart of the West Elk. Allow yourself ample time to return before dark.

Closer to home is the Three Lakes Trail, which departs from the campground. It offers a 3-mile loop hike that extends to the timber line and passes the actual Lost Lake and Dollar Lake. The views of the Beckwiths are better than the fishing on these upper lakes. The fishing at Lost Lake Slough is considerably better to begin with, and is periodically restocked. You can either bank fish or get onto the lake in any hand-propelled craft. No motors are allowed.

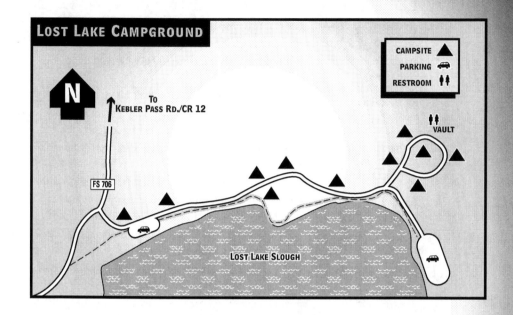

LOST LAKE CAMPGROUND

CAMPSITE ▲
PARKING 🚗
RESTROOM 🚻

N

TO
KEBLER PASS RD./CR 12

VAULT 🚻

FS 706

LOST LAKE SLOUGH

GETTING THERE

From Paonia, drive north on CO 133 to CR 12 (Kebler Pass Road). The sign at the right turn will say "Crested Butte." Turn right on Kebler Pass Road and follow it for 16 miles to FS 706. Turn right on FS 706 and drive 2 more miles to Lost Lake Campground.

GPS COORDINATES

UTM Zone (WGS84)	13S
Easting	0308337
Northing	4304601
Latitude	N 38° 52' 9.8"
Longitude	W 107° 12' 33"

> *Lost Trail is the grandstand of the San Juan Mountains.*

SOMETIMES A LONG DRIVE on a dirt road ends in disappointment, but sometimes you are rewarded for enduring those bumpy, bouncy, dusty rides. In this case, you find Lost Trail Campground. Lost Trail sits in a beautiful valley surrounded on three sides by the San Juans, which form a horseshoe around the headwaters of the Rio Grande, which flow past your tent. Other peaks and crags stand out in bold relief. There are two outstanding hiking areas nearby and two fishing reservoirs close by as well.

The small campground with the big views has only seven campsites spread alongside lower Lost Creek just before its confluence with the Rio Grande. Mostly rock-strewn meadow, Lost Trail has some spruce and aspen that testify to the tough winters up here. The campsites are spread along a rocky road with a vehicle turnaround at the end. Enter the open campground and pass the first campsite on your right. It lies right alongside Lost Trail Creek and has the shade of some spruce. The next site is located in an especially rocky part of the meadow. The next campsite is opposite the creek and is in full-blown open terrain. The views? Simply outstanding. The shade? Nil.

Pass the hand-pump well and the pair of vault toilets for each gender, then come to the auto turnaround. The fifth site is down along the creek far away from the others. If you want privacy, stay here. The sixth site is on a rocky knoll in the center of the turnaround. A few aspens offer scant shade. The last site is away from the creek in the meadow and is an-other site with all view and no shade.

Don't worry too much about privacy—most people who drive this far are going to be like-minded tent campers who want to get way off the beaten track. It's axiomatic: The smaller the campground, the nicer

RATINGS

Beauty: ✿ ✿ ✿ ✿
Privacy: ✿ ✿ ✿
Spaciousness: ✿ ✿ ✿
Quiet: ✿ ✿ ✿ ✿
Security: ✿ ✿ ✿
Cleanliness: ✿ ✿ ✿

campers are to one another. Come here and you'll probably make some new friends.

If (somehow) you tire of taking in the view from the campground, take a hike. The trail system around here is outstanding. The Lost Creek trailhead is just a bit up the road. Here you can take the Lost Creek Trail up to Heart Lake, or go toward the old mining area up toward the Continental Divide. About 30 minutes up the Lost Creek Trail will find you at the junction with the West Lost Creek Trail. Turn left here and come to a giant landslide caused by avalanche activity in 1991. A lake was formed from this event and the Forest Service has stocked it. (And you thought new lakes were only created by man.)

The Continental Divide Trail is farther up Forest Service Road 520 near Stony Pass. This is the easy way to see the high country. The old Beartown mining site is off FS 520 on FS 506. Just down from the campground is the Ute Creek trailhead. After fording the Rio Grande, you can access the Weminuche Wilderness along Ute Creek. This also makes for an isolated fishing experience.

Two nearby reservoirs also offer fishing. Rio Grande Reservoir is closer, but harder to fish on unless you have a boat. It has more than 1,200 surface acres of trout water. Road Canyon Reservoir is a little farther away, however it is much better suited for bank fishing. It has only 140 surface acres, but the shoreline has a gentle grade, parking areas, and spots to put down a chair. The fishing is said to be good.

Bring all you will need to Lost Trail Campground. Supplies are limited in Creede, and you won't have to make an extra trip down that bumpy gravel road.

KEY INFORMATION

ADDRESS:	Lost Trail Campground Divide Ranger District Third and Creede Avenue Creede, CO 81130
OPERATED BY:	USDA Forest Service, Divide Ranger District (Creede)
INFORMATION:	(719) 658-2556; www.fs.fed.us/r2/riogrande
OPEN:	Memorial Day–Labor Day
SITES:	7
EACH SITE HAS:	Picnic table, fire ring
ASSIGNMENT:	First come, first served; no reservation
REGISTRATION:	No registration
FACILITIES:	Pump well, vault toilets
PARKING:	At campsites only
FEE:	No fee
ELEVATION:	9,500 feet
RESTRICTIONS:	*Pets:* On leash only *Fires:* In fire rings only *Alcohol:* At campsites only *Vehicles:* 25 feet *Other:* 14-day stay limit

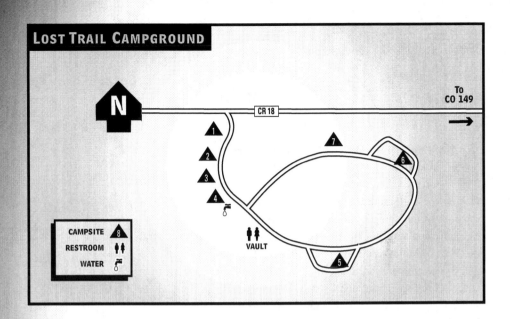

GETTING THERE

From Creede, head west on CO 149 for 20 miles to FS 520 (Rio Grande Reservoir Road) and turn left. Follow FS 520 for 18 miles to Lost Trail Campground, which will be on your left.

GPS COORDINATES

UTM Zone (WGS84)   13S
Easting   0293070
Northing   4182710
Latitude   N 37° 46' 6.0"
Longitude   W 107° 20' 57.0"

45
MESA VERDE
NATIONAL PARK:
MOREFIELD CAMPGROUND

YOU'VE GOT TO SEE MESA VERDE! The sight of the preserved remains of an extinct culture set into the inherent beauty of this park is one of Colorado's finest natural experiences. While driving on the park entrance road you are thinking about cliff dwellings and ancient cultures, but then you look over the Mancos Valley and San Juan scenery and realize that this place is special. The only extraordinary trait of the Morefield campground is its size: more than 400 campsites. It is a pleasant enough place to stay and has adequate amenities to keep you from leaving the mesa, but the park itself has more than enough attractions to make you want to stay longer—the ranger-led tours, the view-laden hiking, darn good auto touring, and high-quality ranger programs every night.

The plethora of campsites are divided into nine loops and are spread out in a basin surrounded by ridges of trees and stone. In the basin, the primary vegetation is the bushy Gambel oak with some occasional piñon pine. Each loop has comfort stations with flush toilets for each gender and combination water fountains/spigots outside them. A community sink area is also within the comfort station.

Pay your fee at the campground entry station and begin looking for a campsite. On the whole, campsite spaciousness is average; privacy depends on the amount of tree cover, which varies considerably. The forest's understory is generally grassy, with some sections of sage and brush. Navajo Loop is popular with tent campers. It is nestled in a hollow off to your left. The loop has many shaded sites and other sites that are exposed to the full sun, which can be tiresome on a long, summer day.

On down the way, Pueblo Road contains three loops and lots of campsites. This area is on a hill and has some piñon pines. The Zuni Loop is the best loop

> *You'll need to stay at least one night at the largest campground in the national-park system to see the cliff dwellings and more at Mesa Verde.*

RATINGS

Beauty: ✪ ✪ ✪
Privacy: ✪ ✪
Spaciousness: ✪ ✪ ✪
Quiet: ✪ ✪ ✪
Security: ✪ ✪ ✪ ✪ ✪
Cleanliness: ✪ ✪ ✪ ✪ ✪

ADDRESS: Mesa Verde National
Park: Morefield
Campground
Aramark Mesa
Verde Company
P.O. Box 277
Mancos, CO 81328

OPERATED BY: Aramark Mesa
Verde

INFORMATION: (970) 564-4300,
(800) 449-2288;
www.visitmesa
verde.com, info
@mesaverde.com

OPEN: Mid-April–October

SITES: 435, some group sites

EACH SITE HAS: Picnic table, fire
grate, tent pads

ASSIGNMENT: For reservations
call (970) 529-4421 or
(800) 449-2288; for
group sites call (970)
533-7731

REGISTRATION: At campground
entry station

FACILITIES: Water spigots, flush
toilets, community
dish sinks, phone
(showers and laun-
dry for fee from con-
cessionaire)

PARKING: At campsites only

FEE: $20 per night,
plus $10 park
entrance fee

ELEVATION: 8,100 feet

RESTRICTIONS: *Pets:* On leash only
Fires: In fire grates
only
Alcohol: At campsites
only
Vehicles: 2 vehicles
per site limit
Other: 14-day stay
limit

up here and has many good tent sites with a variety of sun and shade. There are good views across the basin of Prater Ridge.

Stay away from the Ute Loop. It is the only loop with hookups and is the place of choice for RV campers. The Oraibi, Waipi, and Hano loops are all connected to one another. This area has many camp-sites that take a beating from the sun. The far views are good, but the near views of your fellow campers can be a little too close. The Apache Loop is sometimes closed until the campgrounds begins to fill up. It is similar to the Oraibi loop.

Tent campers share Morefield Campground evenly with RV and pop-up campers. Morefield rarely fills and is fairly quiet, except for summer holidays, especially Memorial Day. A concessionaire offers showers and a laundry for a price. There is also a camp store, gift shop, cafe, and gas station. Snack bars are located at Chapin and Wetherill Mesas. The Far View Lodge, located within the park, offers fine dining. You really can have it all!

Now, the reason why you came—to see the cliff dwellings. You must buy a ticket to go on a ranger-led tour of the three primary dwellings—Long House, Cliff Palace, and Balcony House. Each one was con-structed in the 1200s by the ancestral Pueblos who made their lives atop the "Green Table." Cliff Palace has more than 150 rooms. The ranger leading the tours will satisfy your curiosity about each of the sites. You can tour the Spruce Tree House on your own. All-day and half-day concessionaire guided tours of the park leave Far View Lodge and Morefield camp-ground every morning. Mesa Verde is one place where it is smart to be led around by the nose. You'll want to ask many questions, and these rangers have all the answers.

First check out the park's visitor center and museum to get oriented after setting up camp. You'll come to the campground miles before the visitor center and museum. Make the Chapin Mesa driving tour and see the pit houses that came before the cliff dwellings. View other cliff dwellings from the road. The views of the landscape are exciting too.

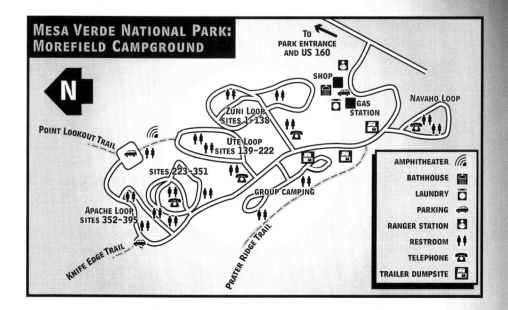

Return to the campground to make the 1.5-mile walk out the Knife Edge to watch the sunset. And for the next day, there is Wetherill Mesa, Prater Ridge, the Cedar Tree Tower, and . . . this place will keep you busy. It is an all-inclusive affair. Bring your camera and a few free days, and have a fulfilling time.

GETTING THERE

From Cortez drive east on US 160 for 7.5 miles to the turnoff for Mesa Verde. Turn right and the Morefield campground is 4 miles on your right.

GPS COORDINATES

UTM Zone (WGS84)	12S
Easting	0723020
Northing	4118670
Latitude	N 37° 11' 16"
Longitude	W 108° 29' 14"

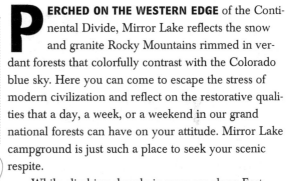

46
MIRROR LAKE
CAMPGROUND

> *Mirror Lake offers a restful alpine setting for tent campers who want to escape the summer heat of the valleys.*

PERCHED ON THE WESTERN EDGE of the Continental Divide, Mirror Lake reflects the snow and granite Rocky Mountains rimmed in verdant forests that colorfully contrast with the Colorado blue sky. Here you can come to escape the stress of modern civilization and reflect on the restorative qualities that a day, a week, or a weekend in our grand national forests can have on your attitude. Mirror Lake campground is just such a place to seek your scenic respite.

While climbing sharply in your car along East Willow Creek, appreciate not only the beauty of the region but the fact that you can access this high lake without having to walk all your supplies in. The road becomes very steep just before arriving at the lake. Make your right turn into the campground and climb another hill. Campsites appear to the left of the road in a stand of spruce, hidden from the water. Then you pop out on a small hill and the lake comes into view. The wind was calm on my visit, and the lake lived up to its name, reflecting Fitzpatrick Peak, Tincup Pass, and Emma Burr Mountain.

What was strange, though, was the state of the campground and lake—they were deserted. Such splendor with only me to appreciate it, although granted, it was a weekday. There were many favorable campsites as I drove through the loop. Several campsites were right on the lake, albeit a bit sun drenched. Others were set off in the woods with partial views of the lake. Though the amenities here are minimal (only vault toilets, you must bring your own water), the perk of easy access to an attractive, high lake right on the divide should attract more campers. The rough road and 16-foot vehicle length limit deters nearly all folks except for determined tent campers. Mirror Lake does get some weekend business, especially later in the summer.

RATINGS

Beauty: ✩ ✩ ✩ ✩
Privacy: ✩ ✩ ✩
Spaciousness: ✩ ✩ ✩
Quiet: ✩ ✩ ✩ ✩
Security: ✩ ✩ ✩
Cleanliness: ✩ ✩ ✩

This same high elevation that lends such beauty also keeps campers from wandering up here in June because of the uncertainty of whether the campground is even open. Call ahead before you make the drive to Mirror Lake.

If you continue forward instead of veering right into the campground, you will come to the boat launch and parking area. The road that traces the left bank of the lake is the rough, four-wheel-drive road over 12,154-foot-high Tincup Pass. Only hand-propelled craft are allowed onto Mirror Lake. It keeps the peace that way. Mirror Lake encompasses 27 acres of clear water that harbors brook and rainbow trout. Forty percent of the bank is fishable; if you bring a raft or canoe you can get to that other sixty percent of shoreline that everyone else misses.

Stream fishers can follow the outlet of Mirror Lake, East Willow Creek. Here, you can catch rainbow, brown, brook, or cutthroat trout. And if you follow East Willow Creek down, you'll come to the big water (and big fish) of Taylor Reservoir. The 2,000-acre lake offers the four fish species described above plus Kokanee salmon, lake trout, and pike. There are boat ramps here as well.

If you don't feel like fishing, take a walk. The four-wheel-drive road up to Tincup Pass is a couple of miles to the top and makes a great day hike. If you prefer, tramp a section of the Timberline Trail. The trailhead is a few hundred yards below the campground. This path generally follows the timber line north below the Sawatch Range. You can take the trail just a mile or so to Garden Basin and an old mine site, or you can walk all the way to Sanford Creek.

Mirror Lake may be best suited for getting an attitude adjustment in an alpine setting, a place to reflect on the really important things in life, like watching the sun set from the top of the Rockies.

KEY INFORMATION

ADDRESS:	Mirror Lake Campground Gunnison Ranger District 216 North Colorado Gunnison, CO 81230
OPERATED BY:	USDA Forest Service, Grand Mesa, Uncompahgre, and Gunnison National Forests
INFORMATION:	(970) 641-0471; www.fs.fed.us/r2/gmug
OPEN:	Mid-June–October
SITES:	10
EACH SITE HAS:	Picnic table, fire ring
ASSIGNMENT:	First come, first served; no reservation
REGISTRATION:	Self-registration on site
FACILITIES:	Vault toilets (no water)
PARKING:	At campsites only
FEE:	$10 per night
ELEVATION:	11,000 feet
RESTRICTIONS:	*Pets:* On leash only *Fires:* In fire rings only *Alcohol:* At campsites only *Vehicles:* 16 feet *Other:* 14-day stay limit

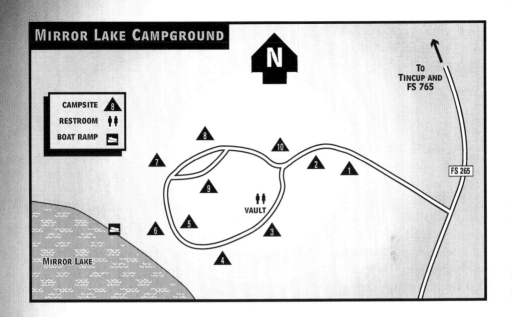

MIRROR LAKE CAMPGROUND

N

TO
TINCUP AND
FS 765

CAMPSITE 8
RESTROOM
BOAT RAMP

FS 265

VAULT

MIRROR LAKE

GETTING THERE

From Almont, drive north on FS 742 (Taylor Canyon Road) for 22 miles to Taylor Reservoir. Turn right at sign for Tincup on FS 765, and follow FS 765 for 8 miles to Tincup. In Tincup, turn left on FS 265 and follow it 3 miles to Mirror Lake.

GPS COORDINATES

UTM Zone (WGS84)   13S
Easting   0375550
Northing   4289720
Latitude   N 38° 44' 51"
Longitude   W 106° 25'55"

47
RIDGWAY STATE
PARK CAMPGROUND

ONE OF THE NEWER **COLORADO** state parks, Ridgway is centered around a 1,000-surface-acre reservoir developed by the Bureau of Reclamation and run by the state of Colorado. This excellently designed recreational area integrates the best in human-made park facilities onto the natural features of the land. Two separate walk-in tent camper areas and three other quality campgrounds make this a must-stop for campers of all stripes.

The Dutch Charlie area features two campgrounds. The Dakota Terraces Campground is on lower, open terrain by the lake and has electrical hookups—this means RVs. The Elk Ridge Campground is high above the lake in a piñon–juniper forest. The views from Elk Ridge of the San Juan and Cimarron mountain ranges will blow your mind. There are two separate loops, both of which have electricity and a surprisingly high number of tent campers. But off Loop D is a set of ten walk-in tent campsites that will appeal to nearly every tent camper.

Walk the paved path that begins the tent-camper loop. The first campsite is handicapped accessible. Beyond that, the gravel path goes beneath some gnarled old piñons, with separate short paths leading to each well-separated site. Three of the sites are near the edge of a precipice over the lake. The mountain view is like a postcard landscape.

All the sites have adequate shade trees, though high noon may present a heat problem. Large, level tent pads make for sound sleeping. Water spigots are located at the tent camper parking area. A modern restroom is nearby, though the showers and laundry are in the campers services building 100 or so yards distant.

Pa-Co-Chu-Puk Campground, 3.5 miles north of the Dutch Charlie area, has two loops that have water, bathrooms, and electricity, but they are out in the open

> *This is one of the finest state parks in Colorado, if not the country.*

RATINGS

Beauty: ✿ ✿ ✿ ✿ ✿
Privacy: ✿ ✿ ✿
Spaciousness: ✿ ✿ ✿ ✿
Quiet: ✿ ✿ ✿ ✿
Security: ✿ ✿ ✿ ✿ ✿
Cleanliness: ✿ ✿ ✿ ✿ ✿

KEY INFORMATION

ADDRESS: Ridgway State Park
28555 US 550
Ridgway, CO 81432

OPERATED BY: Colorado State Parks

INFORMATION: (970) 626-5822;
parks.state.co.us

OPEN: Whole campground
mid-April–
September

SITES: 25 walk-in tent-only
sites, 255 other

EACH SITE HAS: Tent-only has tent
pad, fire grate, grill,
picnic table; others
also have water and
electricity

ASSIGNMENT: By reservation or
pick an available
site on arrival

REGISTRATION: By phone (call (800)
678-CAMP (2267) or
(303) 470-1144 in
Denver)

FACILITIES: Hot showers, flush
toilets, laundry,
phone, vending
machines

PARKING: At campsites or
walk-in tent
campers' parking
area

FEE: $5 Parks Pass plus
$12 per night walk-
in tent site, $16–$20
others

ELEVATION: 7,000 feet Elk Ridge,
6,600 feet Pa-Co-
Chu-Puk

RESTRICTIONS: *Pets:* On leash only
Fires: In fire rings
only
Alcohol: 3.2% beer
only
Vehicles: On paved
roads only
Other: 14-day stay
limit

and full of RVs. However, it also has a 15-site, walk-in tent camping loop that is across the Uncompahgre River from the rest of the park. This loop offers a rustic experience, yet is adjacent to the high-quality facilities that Ridgway offers. This loop is set in a ponderosa pine wood, complemented with Gambel oak and piñon pine, that gently rises up the slope of Log Hill Mesa.

Load your gear on a complimentary cart and bridge the river to the tenters' area. Campsites are snuggled here and there among the trees. The river is clearly audible. At each site, the picnic table and tent pads have been taste-fully leveled, making your experience more comfortable, but still part of nature. Most of the sites are on the outside of the loop and are far from one another, making for a private and uncrowded experience. The water spigot is near the parking area and the showers are a good distance away, by the RV loops.

No matter where you are in this park, the first-rate facilities will make you wish all state parks had $22 million to spend on development. Recreating around here is first rate too. Ridgway Reservoir offers fishing for trout and Kokanee salmon. Waterskiing, parasailing, and riding wave runners are popular. No boat? No problem! The full-service marina will rent you anything from a canoe to a pontoon barge. A swimming beach and playground are ideal for family campers.

The Uncompahgre River flows below the reservoir. You can catch and release fish on the river or keep the fish caught on nearby ponds. Hikers have 15 miles of trails that course through the park to tramp. Four miles of trails are paved for inline skaters and bikers. Ranger-led hikes and programs inform campers about the natural resources of Ridgway. Make sure and check out the visitor center too. The Dallas Creek Recreation Site is at the south end of the park. Here, you can hike and fish along the reservoir and also head up Dallas Creek over the pedestrian bridge.

You would think such a fantastic state park would be constantly full. Not so. However, it does get busy around the major holidays and later in the summer. But I have it on the park manager's word that September is the time to visit Ridgway. Be sure to put this gem of a state park on your to do list.

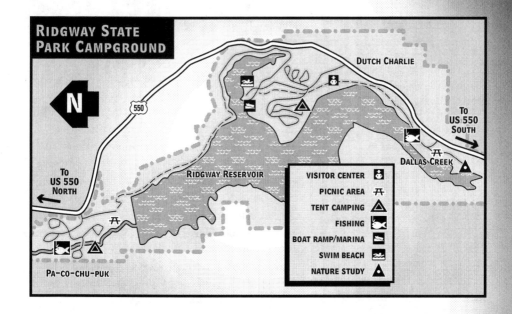

RIDGWAY STATE
PARK CAMPGROUND

N

550

TO
US 550
NORTH

TO
US 550
SOUTH

DUTCH CHARLIE

DALLAS CREEK

RIDGWAY RESERVOIR

PA-CO-CHU-PUK

VISITOR CENTER	
PICNIC AREA	
TENT CAMPING	
FISHING	
BOAT RAMP/MARINA	
SWIM BEACH	
NATURE STUDY	

GETTING THERE

From Ridgway,
drive north on US 550
for 5 miles to the Dutch
Charlie entrance of the park,
which will be on your left.

GPS COORDINATES

UTM Zone (WGS84)	13S
Easting	0260610
Northing	4232460
Latitude	N 38° 12' 28.0"
Longitude	W 107° 44' 3.8"

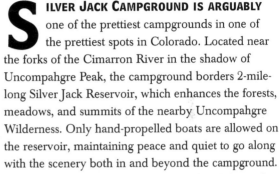

> *Stay among the aspens at the Uncompahgre National Forest's finest campground.*

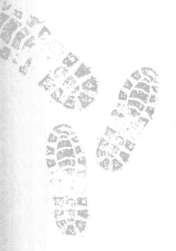

SILVER JACK CAMPGROUND IS ARGUABLY one of the prettiest campgrounds in one of the prettiest spots in Colorado. Located near the forks of the Cimarron River in the shadow of Uncompahgre Peak, the campground borders 2-mile-long Silver Jack Reservoir, which enhances the forests, meadows, and summits of the nearby Uncompahgre Wilderness. Only hand-propelled boats are allowed on the reservoir, maintaining peace and quiet to go along with the scenery both in and beyond the campground.

The campground is situated on a knoll above the lake, surrounded by aspens. Their leaves flutter in the wind, emitting a purr and creating an ever-changing mosaic of light on the forest floor. Tall grass forms an unbroken understory that contrasts with the white trunks of the aspen. This is the reason you come tent camping to begin with.

Silver Jack has three tiered loops. The roads are paved, along with each camper's parking spot, which really cuts down on the dust. The first loop, Ouray, has a short two-way road with campsites along it before the actual loop starts. Ouray is at the lowest level and has 20 campsites set in the aspens. One small meadow breaks up the trees, along with a very occasional small evergreen.

The Chipeta Loop circles around a meadow of its own. Yet all the campsites are in an extremely dense aspen wood. The young trees make for shady campsites and offer great privacy, especially on the upper section of this loop. This seems to be the most popular place to camp.

The Sapinero Loop is the highest on the knoll and is sometimes closed until the campground fills. However, it is my favorite loop. Here, the aspens are older, larger, and allow more light to form a more flowery understory. You can also see the surrounding mountains

RATINGS

Beauty: ✿ ✿ ✿ ✿ ✿
Privacy: ✿ ✿ ✿
Spaciousness: ✿ ✿ ✿
Quiet: ✿ ✿ ✿ ✿
Security: ✿ ✿ ✿ ✿
Cleanliness: ✿ ✿ ✿ ✿ ✿

better. The road rolls upward with campsites spread far apart, though they tighten up as the loop is completed.

Water spigots and vault toilets are evenly spread about the campground. There should be no trouble finding a campsite in June, when the weather is less predictable and can still be chilly. But in July and August, arrive early to ensure a campsite on weekends. September is a great time to visit and watch the aspen leaves change color. Any time is a great time to relax in this wonderful campground setting.

Of course, you may want to get active. Hiking, fishing, and boating are the main activities here. An informal trail circles Silver Jack Reservoir, so you can bank-fish for rainbow trout, brook trout, and Kokanee salmon. By all means, if you have a canoe, bring it. Your arms are the only motor you can use here. The scenery from a boat in the middle of the lake is inspiring. You won't care if you catch fish or not.

Fly fishers like to try their luck on one of the three forks of the Cimarron River, as the waters tumble down from the wilderness above. Beaver Lake lies a mile below Silver Jack and is also popular for fishing. The smaller Fish Creek reservoirs are just a few miles north of Silver Jack on Cimarron Road. No one swims in these chilly lakes.

Silver Jack derived its moniker from the mine of the same name located in the Uncompahgre Wilderness just south of the campground. You can hike up the East Fork Trail (228) to the old mine site. Always be careful near any mine, closed or open. Beyond the mine site are two waterfalls of the East Fork.

You don't have to go to Europe to climb the Matterhorn. There's one right here in the Uncompahgre Wilderness. Take the Middle Fork Trail (227) for a challenging day hike to top the 13,590-foot peak. Uncompahgre Peak is a fourteener, but can't be reached in one day from this side of the wilderness.

For an easier hike, go to Cimarron Ridge, across the reservoir. It can be accessed from Trail 222. You'll end up at 10,800-foot Lou Creek Pass, overlooking your camping paradise. Or hike up to High Mesa on the Alpine Trail, which starts near the campground. Or

KEY INFORMATION

ADDRESS:	Silver Jack Campground Ouray Ranger District 2505 South Townsend Montrose, CO 81402
OPERATED BY:	USDA Forest Service, Grand Mesa, Uncompahgre, and Gunnison National Forests
INFORMATION:	(970) 240-5300; www.fs.fed.us/r2/gmug
OPEN:	Memorial Day–Labor Day
SITES:	60
EACH SITE HAS:	Picnic table, fire grate
ASSIGNMENT:	First come, first served; no reservation
REGISTRATION:	Self-registration on site
FACILITIES:	Water spigots, vault toilets
PARKING:	At campsites only
FEE:	$14 per night
ELEVATION:	8,900 feet
RESTRICTIONS:	*Pets:* On leash only *Fires:* In fire grates only *Alcohol:* At campsites only *Vehicles:* 30 feet *Other:* 14-day stay limit

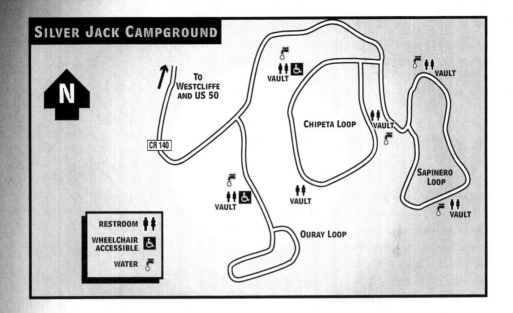

SILVER JACK CAMPGROUND

To WESTCLIFFE AND US 50

CR 140

CHIPETA LOOP

VAULT

VAULT

VAULT

VAULT

SAPINERO LOOP

VAULT

OURAY LOOP

RESTROOM
WHEELCHAIR ACCESSIBLE
WATER

GETTING THERE

From Montrose, drive 23 miles east on US 50 to Cimarron Road. Turn right on Cimarron Road and follow it 21 miles to Silver Jack, which will be on your right.

you may just want to hang out and watch the aspens flutter in the wind.

GPS COORDINATES

UTM Zone (WGS84)   13S
Easting   0277820
Northing   4234830
Latitude   N 38° 14' 2.9"
Longitude   W 107° 32' 17"

49
STONE CELLAR
CAMPGROUND

WHEN YOU CROSS THE Continental Divide at South Pass, Saguache (pronounced suh-WACH) Park opens up before you. It is an expanse of rolling, grassy terrain cut with creeks and bordered by massive peaks fringed in forest land. Smaller, lesser-used forest roads splinter off in all directions, beckoning you to see what lies over the next hill. Farther down, along the Middle Fork of Saguache Creek, lies the Stone Cellar Campground. Beyond the campground, open park land rolls on to the La Garita Mountains and the La Garita Wilderness.

The wilderness looks over (*La Garita* means "the lookout") more meadowlands, as well as old-growth forests and trout-laden streams and lakes. There are more than 120,000 acres and 175 miles of trails to enjoy in this seldom visited slice of wild Colorado. The Wheeler Geologic Area is also within the wilderness. Rock spires, pinnacles, domes, and other stone oddities emerge from the earth.

When you drop down to the campground, you will immediately notice a lack of trees. That's only appropriate because the campground is in Saguache Park. It took a few minutes for me to get used to the openness, but I began to appreciate the scenery: Middle Fork flowing out of a meadow from above into a canyon down below, vertical rock walls rising up at the campground, and the views of the distant mountains.

A wooden stock fence surrounds three of the campsites here. There is one campsite outside the fence a few yards away, toward the head of the meadow on a forest road. This site must either be for campers who have been bad or for campers who love cows, since livestock graze in Saguache Park.

The other three sites border the creek. One site is off to the right and is farthest away from the rock walls. This will avail more views, but less shade. The other

> *Stone Cellar is in the heart of 15,000-acre Saguache Park, the largest meadowland in the entire national forest system.*

RATINGS

Beauty: ✿ ✿ ✿ ✿
Privacy: ✿ ✿
Spaciousness: ✿ ✿ ✿ ✿
Quiet: ✿ ✿ ✿ ✿
Security: ✿ ✿
Cleanliness: ✿ ✿ ✿

ADDRESS: Stone Cellar
Campground
Saguache Ranger
District
46525 CO 114
Saguache, CO 81149

OPERATED BY: USDA Forest
Service, Rio Grande
National Forest

INFORMATION: (719) 655-2547;
www.fs.fed.us/r2/
riogrande

OPEN: Memorial Day–
Labor Day

SITES: 5

EACH SITE HAS: Picnic table, fire ring

ASSIGNMENT: First come,
first served;
no reservation

REGISTRATION: No registration

FACILITIES: Pump well water,
vault toilets

PARKING: At campsites only

FEE: $7 per night

ELEVATION: 9,500 feet

RESTRICTIONS: *Pets:* On leash only
Fires: In fire rings
only
Alcohol: At campsites
only
Vehicles: 25 feet
Other: 14-day stay
limit

two campsites are downstream in a very green, grassy meadow, between a granite wall and the clear, gurgling water. It is a short walk to these campsites from the parking area. A vault toilet and pump well are conveniently set in the middle for all campers, except the site outside the stock fence.

Anyone here should be a tent camper, because if it rains, the road back to CO 114 will be very slick. You shouldn't have a problem unless you are towing something, like a pop-up trailer. If you want to come to Saguache Park but can't stand the thought of camping in the open, several forest roads in the area lead to wooded camp locations. Saguache Park deserves a visit, especially later in the summer when the whole place is awash in wildflowers.

If you do drive the roads around here, make sure to take the marked road to Chimney Rocks. However, to explore the La Garita Wilderness, you must abandon your vehicle and take to your feet. The land is high and the trails start high, then lead even higher.

Farther up Forest Service Road 787 beyond the campground is the South Saguache Trail. It starts at 10,400 feet and follows the creek for good fishing and easy access to the high country toward Half Moon Pass. The Whale Creek Trail starts here too, and heads toward Palmer Mesa.

FS 744, which turns off right before the campground and has the one lonesome campsite, leads farther up the Middle Fork of Saguache Creek to another trailhead. Here you can walk to the headwaters of the Saguache and into lake country. The Half Moon Pass Trail starts here too. It is a 7-mile; one-way hike to the Wheeler Geologic Area, but it can be done in a single day. If you leave early in the morning, you will have time to view the area and still return by nightfall.

The North Fork Saguache has its own trail to headwaters made up of several small tributaries; a few beaver ponds are scattered along the way. This trail is outside the wilderness and can be accessed by FS 776. Walk around or drive around, either way you will get an eyeful at Saguache Park.

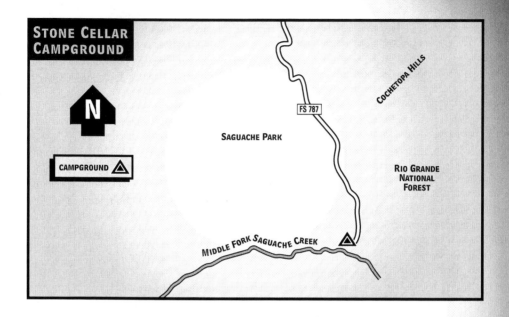

STONE CELLAR CAMPGROUND

N

COCHETOPA HILLS

FS 787

SAGUACHE PARK

RIO GRANDE NATIONAL FOREST

CAMPGROUND ▲

MIDDLE FORK SAGUACHE CREEK

GETTING THERE

From Saguache, head west on CO 114 and follow it 22 miles to FS 804 (Archuleta Creek Road). Turn left on FS 804 and follow it 4 miles to CR NN14. Turn left on CR NN14 and follow it for 0.8 miles to FS 787. Turn right on FS 787 and follow it 13 miles to Stone Cellar Campground.

GPS COORDINATES

UTM Zone (WGS84)   13S
Easting   0352710
Northing   4209340
Latitude   N 38° 1' 12.3"
Longitude   W 106° 40' 42"

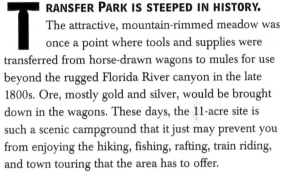

> *Make a transfer to the most attractive campground in the San Juan National Forest.*

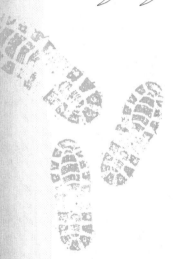

TRANSFER **PARK IS STEEPED IN HISTORY.** The attractive, mountain-rimmed meadow was once a point where tools and supplies were transferred from horse-drawn wagons to mules for use beyond the rugged Florida River canyon in the late 1800s. Ore, mostly gold and silver, would be brought down in the wagons. These days, the 11-acre site is such a scenic campground that it just may prevent you from enjoying the hiking, fishing, rafting, train riding, and town touring that the area has to offer.

Drop into the upper meadow and come to the campground. Miller Mountain stands guard over Transfer Park. There are two camping loops. The right-hand loop has ten campsites and is set in a mature aspen grove mixed with some Ponderosa pine, Douglas fir, and small clearings. Smaller trees and brush form a fairly thick understory. The campsites are large and well separated from one another. Wooden posts delineate the sites from one another. The forest closes near the meadow, then opens back up as the loop is completed. You can find just about any combination of sun and shade you desire. There is one vault toilet and one spigot in the center of the loop.

The left-hand loop is lower and closer to the Florida River. Drop down along Transfer Park and the 15 campsites begin. The forest here is more mixed conifers and thus is shadier. The thicker forest and rock outcrops make for a closed-in, intimate feeling on this loop. The gush of the Florida River can be heard loud and clear. About half the campsites are on the heavily wooded inside of the loop. A few campsites border the river gorge, but a wood fence prevents campers from falling into the river below. Two vault toilets and two water spigots serve this loop.

This campground used to be on a reservation basis, but was taken off because it did not fill. Forest

RATINGS

Beauty: ✿ ✿ ✿ ✿ ✿
Privacy: ✿ ✿ ✿ ✿
Spaciousness: ✿ ✿ ✿ ✿
Quiet: ✿ ✿ ✿ ✿
Security: ✿ ✿ ✿
Cleanliness: ✿ ✿ ✿ ✿

Service personnel say it is rarely at over 50 percent capacity—an odd fact, but a good one, for tent campers who find their way to this gorgeous place.

Those who do make it here now have to choose among the array of nearby activities. You can trace the old mine trail up along the Florida River. It is primarily used now by fishermen who vie for native cutthroat trout and a few Kokanee salmon, which make their way up from Lemon Reservoir. Hiking comes naturally, as the Burnt Timber Trail starts at the top of the campground. This path leads into the nearly 500,000-acre Weminuche Wilderness. A reasonable destination is the southern end of Lime Mesa.

Just up bumpy Forest Service Road 597, which starts by Florida Campground, are two short hikes into Lost Lake and Stump Lake. Lost Lake has no fish. A longer trek goes up Endlich Mesa to the City Reservoir area, which is more attractive than it sounds. Downstream from Transfer Park is Lemon Reservoir. It is a rainbow trout, kokanee salmon, and pike fishery. The popular angling areas are near the dam and at the Lemon Day Use Area.

The rest of the action is down Durango way. It is a historic western town that is cashing in on the tourism craze. The historic district is real, and you can find anything you desire to consume or own. However, if you want to move through some good natural scenery, try the narrow-gauge Silverton Train or a rafting trip on the Piedre or Animas Rivers.

The Durango and Silverton Railroad was constructed in the 1880s to haul gold and silver from the San Juan Mountains. The train trip is an easy way to see the Weminuche Wilderness. It is an all-day affair getting to and from Silverton, but it will be one of the more scenic trips of your life.

The rivers offer more rollicking action. The lower Animas goes through Durango and is a little on the tame side. But the Upper Animas offers Class IV to V rapids. The Piedre has Class III to IV rapids and a wild atmosphere. Contact one of the many outfitters listed at the Durango Chamber of Commerce.

KEY INFORMATION

ADDRESS:	Transfer Park Columbine East Ranger District 367 South Pearl Street Bayfield, CO 81122
OPERATED BY:	USDA Forest Service, San Juan National Forest
INFORMATION:	(970) 884-2512; www.fs.fed.us/r2/sanjuan
OPEN:	Mid-May– Labor Day
SITES:	25
EACH SITE HAS:	Picnic table, fire grate
ASSIGNMENT:	First come, first served; no reservation
REGISTRATION:	Self-registration on site
FACILITIES:	Water spigot, vault toilets, trash pick-up
PARKING:	At campsites only
FEE:	$12 per night
ELEVATION:	8,600 feet
RESTRICTIONS:	*Pets:* On leash only *Fires:* In fire grates only *Alcohol:* At campsites only *Vehicles:* 26 feet *Other:* 14-day stay limit

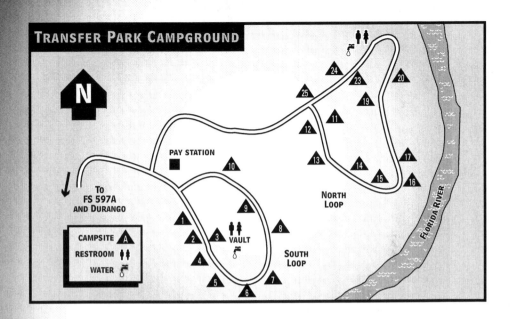

GETTING THERE

From Durango, take CR 240 (Florida Road) north for 14 miles to CR 243. Stay left on CR 243, going for 5 miles, passing Lemon Reservoir, to FS 597A. Turn left on FS 597A and veer left again after crossing the Florida River. Stay right while passing through Florida Campground and come to Transfer Park in 1 mile.

GPS COORDINATES

UTM Zone (WGS84)   13S
Easting   0262990
Northing   4149570
Latitude   N 37° 27' 46.3"
Longitude   W 107° 40' 47"

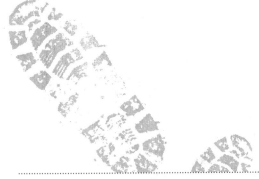
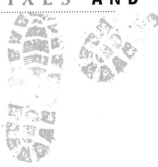

APPENDIXES AND INDEX

APPENDIX A:
CAMPING-EQUIPMENT CHECKLIST

Except for the large and bulky items on this list, we keep a plastic storage container full of the essentials for car camping so they're ready to go when we are. We make a last-minute check of the inventory, resupply anything that's low or missing, and away we go.

COOKING UTENSILS
Bottle opener
Bottles of salt, pepper, spices, sugar, coffee, tea, and cooking oil and maple syrup in water-proof, spillproof containers
Can opener
Corkscrew
Cups, plastic or tin
Dish soap (biodegradable), sponge, and towel
Flatware
Food of your choice
Frying pan, spatula
Fuel for stove
Ice
Lighter, matches in water-proof container
Plates
Pocketknife
Fire starter
Pot with lid
Stove
Tin foil
Wooden spoon

FIRST-AID KIT
Aspirin
Band-Aids
First aid cream
Gauze pads
Insect repellent
Moleskin
Sunscreen/lip balm
Tape, waterproof adhesive

SLEEPING GEAR
Pillow
Sleeping bag
Sleeping pad, inflatable or insulated
Tent with ground tarp and rainfly

MISCELLANEOUS
Bath soap (biodegradable), washcloth, and towel
Camp chair
Candles
Cooler
Deck of cards
Flashlight/headlamp
Paper towels
Plastic zip-top bags

Shovel
Sunglasses
Toilet paper
Warm clothes, raingear, hiking boots
Water bottle
Wool blanket

OPTIONAL
Backpack for hiking
Barbecue grill
Binoculars
Book, novel, magazines
Cell phone
Compass
Field guides on bird, plant, and wildlife identification
Fishing rod and tackle
GPS
Lantern
Maps (road, trail, topographic, etc.)

APPENDIX B:
CONTACT INFORMATION

U.S. BUREAU OF LAND MANAGEMENT

Big Dominguez Campground
2815 H Road
Grand Junction, CO 81506
(970) 244-3000
www.co.blm.gov/gjra/dominguezcg.htm

Little Snake BLM Field Office
455 Emerson Street
Craig, CO 81625
(970) 826-5087 or (970) 826-5000;
www.co.blm.gov/lsra/camping.htm

COLORADO STATE PARKS

Arkansas Headwater Recreation Area
307 West Sackett Avenue, P.O. Box 126
Salida, CO 81201
(719) 539-7289; parks.state.co.us

Bonny Lake State Park
30010 County Road 3
Idalia, CO 80735
(970) 354-7306; parks.state.co.us
bonny.lake.park@state.co.us;
Bonny marina and store: (970) 354-7339

Colorado State Forest
2746 Jackson County Road 41
Walden, CO 80480
(970) 723-8366; parks.state.co.us;
state_forest@state.co.us

Golden Gate Canyon State Park
92 Crawford Gulch Road
Golden, CO 80403
(303) 582-3707 or (303) 642-3856 in
summer; parks.state.co.us
golden.gate.park@state.co.us

Jackson Lake State Park
26363 CR 3
Orchard, CO 80649
(970) 645-2551; parks.state.co.us
jackson.lake@state.co.us

Mueller State Park Campground
P.O. Box 39
Divide, CO 80814
(719) 687-2366; parks.state.co.us
mueller.park@state.co.us

Ridgway State Park
28555 Highway 550
Ridgway, CO 81432
(970) 626-5822; parks.state.co.us

Rifle Falls State Park Campground
00050 Road 219
Rifle, CO 81650
(970) 625-1607
parks.state.co.us
rifle.gap.park@state.co.us

Steamboat Lake State Park Campground
Box 750
Clark, CO 80428
(970) 879-3922; parks.state.co.us/
steamboat; steamboat@state.co.us

**Larimer County Parks and Open Lands
   Department**
1800 South County Road 31
Loveland, CO 80537
970) 679-4570
www.larimer.org/parks

APPENDIX B:
CONTACT
INFORMATION
(continued)

NATIONAL PARK SERVICE

Colorado National Monument
Fruita, CO 81521
(970) 858-3617; www.nps.gov/colm

Curecanti National Recreation Area
102 Elk Creek
Gunnison, CO 81230
(970) 641-2337 ext. 205; www.nps.gov/cure

Dinosaur National Monument
4545 East Highway 40
Dinosaur, CO 81610-9724
(970) 374-3000 or (435) 781-7700;
www.nps.gov/dino

Great Sand Dunes National Monument
11999 Highway 150
Mosca, CO 81146
(719) 378-2312; www.nps.gov/grsa

North Rim Campground
102 Elk Creek
Gunnison, CO 81230
(970) 641-2337; www.nps.gov/blca

Rocky Mountain National Park
Estes Park, CO 80517
(970) 586-1206; www.nps.gov/romo

USDA FOREST SERVICE:
ARAPAHO AND ROOSEVELT
NATIONAL FORESTS,
PAWNEE NATIONAL GRASSLAND

Boulder Ranger District
2140 Yarmouth Avenue
Boulder, CO 80301
(303) 541-2500; www.fs.fed.us/r2/arnf

Canyon Lakes Ranger District
2150 Centre Avenue, Building E
Fort Collins, CO 80526
(970) 295-6700; www.fs.fed.us/r2/arnf

Pawnee National Grassland
660 "O" Street
Greeley, CO 80631
(970) 346-5000; www.fs.fed.us.r2/arnf

Sulphur Ranger District
9 Ten Mile Drive, P.O. Box 10
Granby, CO 80446
(970) 887-4100

USDA FOREST SERVICE:
DIVIDE RANGER DISTRICT

Divide Ranger District
3rd and Creede Avenue
Creede, CO 81130
(719) 658-2556; www.fs.fed.us/r2/riogrande

APPENDIX B:
CONTACT
INFORMATION
(continued)

USDA FOREST SERVICE:
GRAND MESA, UNCOMPAHGRE, AND
GUNNISON NATIONAL FORESTS

Grand Valley Ranger District
277 Crossroads Boulevard, Suite A
Grand Junction, CO 81506
(970) 242-8211; **www.fs.fed.us/r2/gmug**

Gunnison Ranger District
216 North Colorado
Gunnison, CO 81230
(970) 641-0471; **www.fs.fed.us/r2/gmug**

Ouray Ranger District
2505 South Townsend
Montrose, CO 81402
(970) 240-5300; **www.fs.fed.us/r2/gmug**

Paonia Ranger District
P.O. Box 1030
North Rio Grande Avenue
Paonia, CO 81428
(970) 527-4131; **www.fs.fed.us/r2/gmug**

USDA FOREST SERVICE:
MEDICINE BOW–ROUTT NATIONAL
FORESTS, THUNDER BASIN NATIONAL
GRASSLAND
Yampa Ranger District
P.O. Box 7, 300 Roselawn Avenue
Yampa, CO 80483
(970) 638-4516; **www.fs.fed.us/r2/mbr**

USDA FOREST SERVICE: PIKE AND SAN
ISABEL NATIONAL FORESTS, CIMARRON
AND COMANCHE NATIONAL GRASSLANDS

Grand Valley Ranger District
325 West Rainbow Boulevard
Salida, CO 81201
(970) 242-8211; **www.fs.fed.us/r2/psicc/sal**

Leadville Ranger District
810 Front Street
Leadville, CO 80461
(719) 486-0749
www.fs.fed.us/r2/psicc/leadville

San Carlos Ranger District
3170 East Main Street
Cañon City, CO 81212
(719) 269-8500;
www.fs.fed.us/r2/psicc/sanc

South Platte Ranger District
19316 Goddard Ranch Court
Morrison, CO 80465
(303) 275-5610; **www.fs.fed.us/r2/psicc/spl**

USDA FOREST SERVICE:
RIO GRANDE NATIONAL FOREST

Cathedral Campground
Divide Ranger District
13308 West Highway 160
Del Norte, CO 81132
(719) 657-3321; **www.fs.fed.us/r2/riogrande**

APPENDIX B:
CONTACT
INFORMATION
(continued)

USDA FOREST SERVICE:
RIO GRANDE NATIONAL FOREST *(continued)*

Conejos Peak Ranger District
15571 County Road T-5
La Jara, CO 81140
(719) 274-8971; **www.fs.fed.us/r2/riogrande**

Saguache Ranger District
46525 CO 114
Saguache, CO 81149
(719) 655-2547; **www.fs.fed.us/r2/riogrande**

USDA FOREST SERVICE:
SAN JUAN NATIONAL FOREST

Mancos-Dolores Ranger District
100 North 6th Street
Dolores, CO 81323
(970) 882-7296; **www.fs.fed.us/r2/sanjuan**

Pagosa Ranger District
108 Second Street
Pagosa Springs, CO 81147
(970) 264-2268; **www.fs.fed.us/r2/sanjuan**

Transfer Park Columbine East
   Ranger District
367 South Pearl Street
Bayfield, CO 81122
(970) 884-2512; **www.fs.fed.us/r2/sanjuan**

USDA FOREST SERVICE:
WHITE RIVER NATIONAL FOREST

Blanco Ranger District
317 East Market Street
Meeker, CO 81641
(970) 878-4039
www.fs.fed.us/r2/whiteriver

Eagle Ranger District
P.O. Box 720, 125 West Fifth Street
Eagle, CO 81631
(970) 328-6388
www.fs.fed.us/r2/whiteriver

Holy Cross Ranger District
24747 US 24
Minturn, CO 81645
(970) 827-5715; **www.wildernet.com**

INDEX

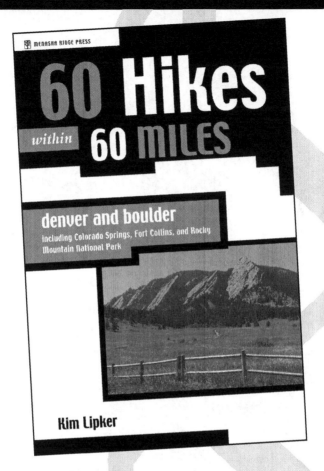

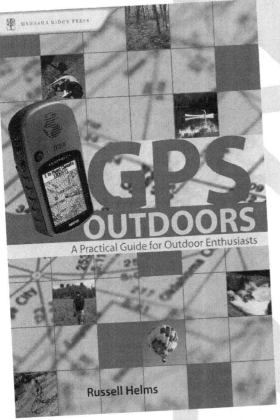

GPS OUTDOORS

by Russell Helms
ISBN 10: 0-89732-967-8
ISBN 13: 978-0-89732-967-5
$10.95
120pages

Whether you're a hiker on a weekend trip through the Great Smokies, a backpacker cruising the Continental Divide Trail, a mountain biker kicking up dust in Moab, a paddler running the Lewis and Clark bicentennial route, or a climber pre-scouting the routes up Mount Shasta, a simple handheld GPS unit is fun, useful, and can even be a lifesaver.

DEAR CUSTOMERS AND FRIENDS,

SUPPORTING YOUR INTEREST IN OUTDOOR ADVENTURE, travel, and an active lifestyle is central to our operations, from the authors we choose to the locations we detail to the way we design our books. Menasha Ridge Press was incorporated in 1982 by a group of veteran outdoorsmen and professional outfitters. For 25 years now, we've specialized in creating books that benefit the outdoors enthusiast.

Almost immediately, Menasha Ridge Press earned a reputation for revolutionizing outdoors- and travel-guidebook publishing. For such activities as canoeing, kayaking, hiking, backpacking, and mountain biking, we established new standards of quality that transformed the whole genre, resulting in outdoor-recreation guides of great sophistication and solid content. Menasha Ridge continues to be outdoor publishing's greatest innovator.

The folks at Menasha Ridge Press are as at home on a white-water river or mountain trail as they are editing a manuscript. The books we build for you are the best they can be, because we're responding to your needs. Plus, we use and depend on them ourselves.

We look forward to seeing you on the river or the trail. If you'd like to contact us directly, join in at www.trekalong.com or visit us at www.menasharidge.com. We thank you for your interest in our books and the natural world around us all.

SAFE TRAVELS,

BOB SEHLINGER
PUBLISHER

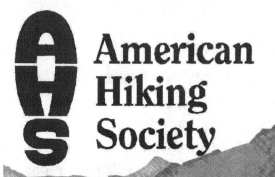
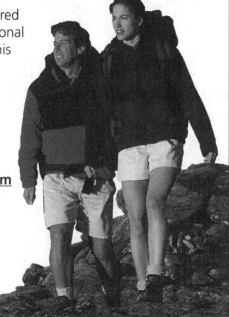
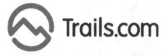